The short guide to health and social care

Jon Glasby

D0731461

First edition published in Great Britain in 2019 by

Policy Press
University of Bristol
1-9 Old Park Hill
Bristol BS2 8BB
UK
+44 (0)117 954 5940
pp-info@bristol.ac.uk
www.policypress.co.uk

North America office:
Policy Press
c/o The University of Chicago Press
1427 East 60th Street
Chicago, IL 60637, USA
t: +1 773 702 7700
f: +1 773-702-9756
sales@press.uchicago.edu
www.press.uchicago.edu

© Policy Press 2019

British Library Cataloguing in Publication Data
A catalogue record for this book is available from the British Library.

Library of Congress Cataloging-in-Publication Data
A catalog record for this book has been requested.

ISBN 978-1-4473-5058-3 paperback
ISBN 978-1-4473-5060-6 ePub
ISBN 978-1-4473-5061-3 Mobi
ISBN 978-1-4473-5247-1 ePdf

The right of Jon Glasby to be identified as the author of this work has been asserted by him in accordance with the Copyright, Designs and Patents Act 1988.

Every reasonable effort has been made to obtain permission to reproduce copyrighted material. If, however, anyone knows of an oversight, please contact the publisher.

All rights reserved: no part of this publication may be reproduced, stored in a retrieval system, or transmitted in any form or by any means, electronic, mechanical, photocopying, recording, or otherwise without the prior permission of Policy Press.

The statements and opinions contained within this publication are solely those of the author and not of the University of Bristol or Policy Press. The University of Bristol and Policy Press disclaim responsibility for any injury to persons or property resulting from any material published in this publication.

Policy Press works to counter discrimination on grounds of gender, race, disability, age and sexuality.

Cover design by Qube Design Associates, Bristol
Printed and bound in Great Britain by CMP, Poole
Policy Press uses environmentally responsible print partners

Contents

List of boxes

Concepts and Debates

Facts and Figures

Key Sources

Voices of Experience

Acknowledgements

A big thank you to everyone at Policy Press (especially Catherine Gray and Alison Shaw for proposing this book and helping to develop its focus and contribution). Depending on how you count it (edited collections, series editing, multiple editions etc), this is my 20th book with Policy Press – and every single one has been a privilege! I'm also really grateful to colleagues at the University of Birmingham's Health Services Management Centre and Department of Social Work and Social Care, who have helped me with advice, ideas and resources.

The author and publisher would like to thank the following for permission to reproduce copyright material: Age UK for extracts on pages 64–65; Bob Hudson and the London School of Economics British Politics and Policy blog for extracts on page 49–51; Community Care for extracts on pages 57–58; Nuffield Trust for the figure on page 29; Peoplehub for extracts on pages 69–71; Pulse and Dominique Thompson for extracts on pages 136–137; and Yvonne Sawbridge for extracts on pages 83–84.

Glossary

The following terms and concepts are set out in **bold** in the main body of the text (when they are used substantively rather than just in passing).

assets–based approaches   rather than focusing on what people can't do for themselves or need help with, assets-based approaches look at people's strengths and networks, and try to build on these

best value   moving on from compulsory competitive tendering, councils have a duty to secure best value when deciding how services should be provided (so they should be contracted out if this will be better than delivering them in-house)

Beveridge Report   official report published in 1942 and influential in the subsequent welfare reforms of the 1940s and beyond (often seen as the founding document of the UK welfare state)

capping   government limits on the amounts by which local councils can increase local taxes

Care Act 2014   key legislation consolidating and reforming adult social care

care closer to home   policies over time which have sought to move care out of specialist settings (such as hospitals) into the community or people's own homes

care manager/management   new title for social workers following the community care reforms of the early 1990s (incorporating language from the private sector, with social workers now seen as the 'managers' of people's care)

care package   a set of services commissioned by social workers/ care managers to meet a person's assessed needs

care plan   sets out a person's assessed needs and the care package that will help meet these needs

Clinical Commissioning Groups (CCGs)   in England, general practitioner (GP)-led CCGs decide what health services are needed locally and purchase these from a range of different providers

commissioning   a process of assessing the needs of a local area, deciding what services will meet those needs, securing those services from a range of different providers, monitoring quality and evaluating outcomes. Separating commissioning from provision is also described as a purchaser-provider split

community care reforms   a series of changes to adult social work and to the funding of care homes in the early 1990s, trying to promote care closer to home. Social workers are now care managers, responsible for assessing needs and drawing up a care package of services to meet these needs

compulsory competitive tendering   requirement for local councils to put a range of services out to the market to see if other providers could offer the same service for less money

direct payments   cash payments to people with social care needs instead of directly provided services (so that the person can hire their own personal assistants or buy care from an independent sector provider). With the right support, this can give greater choice and control. Direct payments have since been extended to some forms of health care

double-bed relationship   recognition that the state needs doctors to deliver health care, and that doctors have to work with the state given it is the main funder of health care

Emergency Medical Service   state-run hospital services set up during the Second World War and contributing to the subsequent creation of the NHS

emotional labour   a recognition that care work can be extremely emotionally distressing, and that we need to find ways to support frontline staff in the work they do, and to keep ourselves emotionally healthy

empowerment   an approach which seeks to share power between health and social care professionals and people using services

Foundation Trusts   NHS Trusts (initially high-performing Trusts) who – in theory – have been given a degree of additional freedom and flexibility from central control

free personal care   introduced in Scotland, so that people in care homes receive help with activities of daily living (washing, dressing, eating) free of charge (in the same way as such care in a hospital would be free), but make a financial contribution towards their living and accommodation costs

Friends and Family Test   a mechanism to ask patients whether they would recommend a particular health service to their friends or family (there is also a version asking staff whether they would recommend their own service)

gearing   ensuring that local councils can't increase spending by too much by ensuring that the bulk of any increase falls on politically unpopular local taxes and/or user charges

general management   introduced in the NHS from the early 1980s as a way of incorporating lessons from the commercial sector and improving the quality of care by having leaders with managerial rather than necessarily clinical skills responsible for the delivery of health services

Gross Domestic Product (GDP)   a measure of the strength of a country's economy

health inequalities   people from higher socioeconomic backgrounds tend to have access to more resources and better health than people from less privileged backgrounds

Health and Wellbeing Boards   committees (in England) responsible for assessing the needs of the local area, devising a strategy to meet these needs and joining up health and social care

independent living   a movement of disabled people arguing for a social model of disability and that disabled people should have the same choice and control over their lives as non-disabled people

intermediate care   services which are designed to prevent people in a crisis (usually older people) from being admitted to hospital, or to facilitate swift discharge from hospital (might include rapid response nursing services, short-term rehabilitation and step-up/step-down beds in care homes for people to have a short stay either side of a hospital admission)

internal market   creation of competition between NHS providers as a way of trying to improve the quality and responsiveness of services

medical model of disability   a focus on disability as a
biological problem with the individual (see below for the social
model of disability)

micro-enterprise   more common in social care, these are very
small businesses (perhaps 1–5 members of staff, sometimes just a
sole trader) providing care and support to a very small number of
people, often set up by people with personal experience of care
services and with scope to be more flexible, innovative and close
to the person being supported due to their very small size

mixed economy of care   services provided by a range of
public, private and voluntary organisations

National Assistance Act 1948   ended the Poor Law and
created a new system which separated practical support with
care needs (social care) from support for those in poverty (social
security)

National Health Service Act 1946   created the NHS (which
began life two years later in 1948)

NHS Constitution   a government document setting out key
values, rights and expectations for patients, the public and NHS
staff

NHS mandate   objectives agreed between the government and
NHS England as to what health services will try to prioritise and
achieve during the subsequent year

NHS Trust   Hospital, mental health and community health
services in England are delivered by freestanding 'Trusts', who
are commissioned to deliver particular services to the local
population. They are modelled in part on private companies, with
a Board of Directors and a Chair

Non-Executive Directors   the Boards of NHS Trusts are
made up of a mix of Executives (who run the organisation on a
day-to-day basis) and Non-Executives (who act as critical friends
to the organisation and try to make sure that decisions are made
in a good way by asking challenging questions)

parity of esteem   a policy commitment to trying to ensure that
mental health services are treated as an equal priority to physical
health services

patient choice   approach to organising health care whereby
patients can choose where they receive their care, with the money
following the patient (so that 'good' providers attract more
patients and receive more funding, in theory at least)

Payment by Results   national payment system (in England) so
that hospitals and other providers are paid a set amount of money
for each person they see and the different interventions they
provide

personal budgets   beginning in social care, this involves
deciding how much money is available to spend on meeting
someone's assessed needs, and then giving the person much
greater say over how this money is spent on their behalf (and
over how much control the person wants to have over the money
itself). This might range from receiving a direct payment to a
social worker/council managing the money on someone's behalf
(but with the person able to exercise greater choice and control
over what the money is used for). This has since been extended
into parts of the NHS

personalisation agenda   a broader approach which tries to
tailor individual services to the needs of the individual and to
enable people to have greater choice and control (often associated
with assets-based approaches, direct payments and personal
budgets)

Poor Law   the system for supporting those in poverty from Tudor times up to the Second World War

purchaser-provider split   separating the provision of services from the body responsible for deciding what is needed/who is best to provide such services. This created an internal/quasi-market in the NHS and is associated with the use of choice and competition as a mechanism for trying to improve care

quasi-market   when market mechanisms were introduced into health and social care, it was recognised that these aren't full markets in a traditional sense (we often don't buy our care directly, but have a third party – a local council or a Clinical Commissioning Group – to commission our care on our behalf)

reablement   an attempt to refocus home care services by providing intensive six-week support/rehabilitation after a period in hospital or some sort of crisis to help an older person regain skills and as much independence as possible

social construction   the ways in which social practices and cultural assumptions create and reinforce ideas until they seem to be natural and inevitable, even though they are the product of human activity that could be changed. (For example, 'sex' is about biological differences between men and women, while 'gender' is to do with the roles we assume that men and women may undertake; the latter is 'socially constructed')

social determinants of health   the way in which our health is shaped by the position we occupy within the society in which we live and the way society is organised

social divisions   the ways we tend to divide groups of people up on the basis of sex, ethnicity, age, sexuality and other social characteristics (and the assumptions, stereotypes and discrimination that this can lead to)

social enterprise   an organisation that generates funds in a more commercial manner, but uses this to deliver social ends (sometimes seen as a cross between the altruism of some public/voluntary sector organisations and the commercial skills and entrepreneurialism of some private organisations)

social model of disability   developed by disabled people themselves, this approach sees disability as arising out of the way in which society discriminates against people with impairments (and therefore focuses primarily on trying to change society rather than trying to 'cure' the individual). See social constructionism

Sustainability and Transformation Plans/Partnerships (STPs)   shared plans to reconfigure health services across 44 areas of England, seen by many as attempt to overcome the fragmentation of the 2012 Lansley reforms without a major national reorganisation or new legislation

tripartite system   key element of the design of the early NHS, with separate systems for hospitals, community health services and general practice (with fragmentation an ongoing and current risk)

user involvement   a commitment to seeking the experience and ideas of people using health and social services to improve care and shape future provision

Other abbreviations and jargon

In spite of the glossary above, health and social care remain full of abbreviations, acronyms and jargon (and these change over time as new policies are introduced, as services are reorganised and as new concepts become suddenly popular). This is helpfully acknowledged by NHS England: 'when you are new to working with the NHS it can be difficult to get used to some of the language and terms that are used' (www.england.nhs.uk/participation/resources/involvejargon/). To help, it signposts people to:

• An 'acronym buster' provided by the NHS Confederation (a membership body for NHS organisations planning, funding or providing care): www.nhsconfed.org/acronym-buster
• A care and support 'jargon buster' provided by Think Local Act Personal (a partnership of more than 50 organisations committed to transforming health and care through personalisation and community-based support): www.thinklocalactpersonal.org.uk/Browse/Informationandadvice/CareandSupportJargonBuster

Introduction: why health and social care matter

The NHS belongs to the people. It is there to improve our health and wellbeing, supporting us to keep mentally and physically well, to get better when we are ill and, when we cannot fully recover, to stay as well as we can to the end of our lives. It works at the limits of science – bringing the highest levels of human knowledge and skill to save lives and improve health. It touches our lives at times of basic human need, when care and compassion are what matter most. (NHS, 2015, p 2)

Social work in its various forms addresses the multiple, complex transactions between people and their environments. Its mission is to enable all people to develop their full potential, enrich their lives, and prevent dysfunction. Professional social work is focused on problem solving and change. As such, social workers are change agents in society and in the lives of the individuals, families and communities they serve. (British Association of Social Workers, 2014, p 6)

As this book was being written during late 2017/early 2018, the challenges of delivering health and social care in a difficult policy and financial context were seldom far from the front pages of the papers. In November 2017, the Chief Executive of NHS England, Simon Stevens, made a very strong public statement about the funding the NHS needed to continue delivering current standards of care, and made it clear that ongoing underfunding would have to lead to difficult conversations about what the NHS could afford to provide in future. This was greeted with a furious reaction from Downing Street and the Chancellor, with suggestions in the media that the NHS had previously been given what it had asked for, that they saw Stevens as personally responsible for the extent to which the NHS could successfully manage the winter (or not) and that more funding would have been given to the health service had it not been for these very public demands for more money. As winter progressed, hospitals were under extreme pressure, and a number of senior doctors wrote to the Prime Minister to say that the NHS was in crisis and that patients were dying in hospital corridors.

At the same time, there was widespread debate about the future funding of social care services for older people – the mishandling of which had been instrumental in the Conservatives' disastrous performance in the snap election they called in May 2017. Critics pointed out that another debate about these issues was unnecessary given they had been reviewed and discussed at length on at least 12 previous occasions since 1999 and each time kicked into the long grass for someone else to sort out in future. Cash-strapped councils also pointed out that they were in financial crisis now and could not wait for a long-term solution – and many were dismayed that the 2017 Budget did not even seem to mention adult social care. Others pointed out that a pledge to reform social care for older people made little mention of carers, and excluded services for disabled people of working age, people with mental health problems and people with learning disabilities. There was also widespread concern that discussion would be dominated by pressures on the health service rather than looking at social care in its entirety and as an important service in its own right.

Throughout this period, the headlines were stark – and became even bleaker over time and as winter hit (see **Voices of Experience 1**).

Voices of Experience 1: Health and social care in the headlines (2017–18)

'Exceptional' NHS Wales winter pressure days *(BBC)*

Government accused of 'dragging their feet' on social care funding shake-up: Ministers delay publication of social care green paper until summer 2018, prompting claims they are 'kicking the can down the road' *(Independent)*

Without a clear strategy, adult social care will continue to lurch from crisis to crisis *(Guardian)*

Scotland's NHS 'brain drain' as nurses quit to work overseas *(Express)*

NHS budget plan not enough, say bosses *(BBC)*

Now is not the time for a fight with Treasury, NHS boss Simon Stevens told *(The Times)*

Crisis as thousands of nurses quit NHS due to high workloads and low pay *(Metro)*

NHS crisis: Overworked Northern Ireland nurses in tears and patients with no hope of being seen *(Belfast Telegraph)*

Care workers 'exhausted' by staff shortage *(BBC Northern Ireland)*

NHS 'workforce crisis' sees 1,600 GPs quit since health bosses pledged to tackle shortages *(Sun)*

Patients 'dying in hospital corridors' *(BBC)*

Health service to face 'worst winter in history' *(Express)*

Budget 2017: NHS trusts given extra £350m for entire winter, despite Brexit bus promising £350m a week *(Independent)*

Theresa May tells NHS boss he will be accountable for winter performance *(Guardian)*

This was just a snapshot at a particular moment in time, but all this matters for at least three key reasons:

1. Millions of people use health and social services each year (see **Facts and Figures 1**), and these can be quite literally a matter of life and death. When services work well, lives are saved, transformed and enriched. When care is poor or non-existent, people can die, lives are blighted, and people suffer. When things go wrong, there can be physical harm, but the emotional and psychological impact can be just as severe and often lasts longer. It is hard to imagine a topic more important than health and social care, because these matter so much to so many people.

2. Because of this, both health and social care (but particularly the NHS) receive large amounts of public funding – and this makes what they do and how well they are perceived to do it inherently political. In previous years, we have seen individual politicians accosted in public for individual failings in care, and – no matter whether it is fair to hold one individual to account for one particular incident or situation in such a complex system – the reality is we often do see politicians as personally and directly responsible for what happens in frontline services. More generally, the sheer amount of public money we devote to health and social care, as well as the overriding importance of such services for us all, means that politicians, the media and the public all have strong views on current care and what should happen next.

3. Although less visible, health and social care have a key economic role, whether through the individual spending of a huge workforce, the goods and services which health and social care organisations buy, or the impact of having a fit and healthy workforce. When people are physically or mentally unwell, or when they have unmet care needs that prevent them from working, we have a smaller potential workforce, higher social security spending, more absences from work and reduced productivity. While health and social care spending is often seen as something of a bottomless pit, it could also be viewed as a form of investment in creating a healthy society and a healthy economy.

Nor are these issues confined to the UK. At the time of writing, the US was mired in controversy over attempts by Donald Trump to reverse the health care reforms of his predecessor, Barack Obama. Parts of Canada were debating how best to ensure that frail older people who are medically fit to leave hospital can be supported in the community rather than remaining in hospital for prolonged periods. Australia was introducing a new national disability insurance scheme, while China was grappling with how to improve health care in rural areas and how to respond to the needs of a rapidly ageing society. In 2016, public health experts across South America, the Caribbean and beyond debated how best to respond to the Zika virus, while 2013–16 witnessed the devastation caused in West Africa and elsewhere by the Ebola virus. As the UK prepared for winter in 2017, its planning was influenced by awareness of Australia's recent flu epidemic, with fears that 2017–18 might prove particularly challenging for the UK too.

Of course, many of these issues play out differently in different national contexts and cultures – and much depends on national politics, economics and society. For example, US debates seem to have been as much about different beliefs around the role of the state in ensuring health care needs are met, and attitudes to this are very different in the US compared to the UK. However, while the specifics of health and social care policy and practice are often unique to a particular national context, many of the themes addressed in this book are international and universal. Irrespective of where we live and what kind of system we have, all of us will be born, grow older and die, and many of us will have health problems and need some form of practical care and assistance en route. How good our health and social care are, and how these systems work, are therefore crucial issues for all of us.

Facts and Figures 1: Health and social care in numbers

The NHS: size and activity

Each year, organisations such as the NHS Confederation produce helpful overviews of NHS statistics (often focused on England, but with links to similar data for other parts of the UK):

- *The NHS deals with over 1 million patients every 36 hours.*
- *In 2015/16 there were 40% more operations completed by the NHS compared to 2005/06, with an increase from 7.215m to 10.119m.*
- *There were 16.252m total hospital admissions in 2015/16, 28% more than a decade earlier (12.679m).*
- *Total annual attendances at Accident & Emergency departments were 23.372m in 2016/17, 23.5% higher than a decade earlier (18.922m).*
- *In real terms the budget is expected to increase from £120.512bn in 2016/17 to £123.202bn by 2019/20. Despite this, the NHS net deficit for the 2015/16 financial year was £1.851 billion.*
- *In March 2017, the NHS employed (full-time equivalent): 106,430 doctors; 285,893 nurses and health visitors; 21,597 midwives; 132,673 scientific, therapeutic and technical staff; 19,772 ambulance staff; 21,139 managers; and 9,974 senior managers. In March 2017 there were 33,423 full-time equivalent GPs, which is a reduction of 890 (2.59%) on March 2016.*

Source: NHS statistics, facts and figures, NHS Confederation, www. nhsconfed.org/resources/key-statistics-on-the-nhs

The NHS in an international context

- In comparison with the health care systems of ten other countries (Australia, Canada, France, Germany, The Netherlands, New Zealand, Norway, Sweden, Switzerland and USA), the NHS was found to be the most impressive overall by the Commonwealth Fund in 2017. The NHS was rated as the best system in terms of safe care, affordability and equity. It was also ranked first in the 'care process' category, which encompassed preventative care, safe care, coordinated care and engagement, and patient preferences.

- Health expenditure in the UK was 9.75% of GDP in 2016. This compares to 17.21% in the USA, 11.27% in Germany, 10.98% in France, 10.50% in the Netherlands, 10.37% in Denmark, 10.34% in Canada, 8.98% in Spain and 8.94% in Italy.

- Expenditure per capita for the UK was the equivalent of $4,192 in 2016, compared to $9,892 in the USA, $5,551 in Germany, $5,385 in the Netherlands, $5,199 in Denmark, $4,644 in Canada, $4,600 in France, $3,391 in Italy and $3,248 in Spain.

- The UK had 2.8 physicians per 1,000 people in 2016, compared to 4.1 in Germany, 3.9 in Spain, 3.8 in Italy, 3.5 in Australia, 3.4 in France, 3.0 in New Zealand and 2.7 in Canada.

- The UK had 2.6 hospital beds per 1,000 people in 2015, compared to 8.1 in Germany, 6.1 in France, 3.2 in Italy, 3.0 in Spain, 2.8 in the USA, 2.7 in New Zealand and 2.6 in Denmark.

Source: NHS statistics, facts and figures, NHS Confederation, www.nhsconfed.org/resources/key-statistics-on-the-nhs

Social care: size and activity

Perhaps because it is organised on a more local level, it is harder to find a simple overview for adult social care. However:

- In 2014, the National Audit Office (NAO) estimated that spending on adult social care arranged by local authorities was £19 billion (with £2.5 billion of this paid in service user contributions). People funding their own care contributed another £10 billion. There were around 1.5 million people working in adult social care, and over 5 million unpaid carers providing informal care to the value of £100 billion per year.
- Rising need and demand coupled with significant financial cuts in local government have led to increasing pressures on adult social care budgets, informal carers and the NHS. As the NAO concluded (2014, p 11):

  Pressures on the care system are increasing. Providing adequate adult social care poses a significant public service challenge and there are no easy answers. People are living longer and some have long-term and complex health conditions that require managing through care. Need for care is rising while public spending is falling, and there is unmet need. Departments do not know if we are approaching the limits of the capacity of the system to continue to absorb these pressures.

- In 2016, there were around 20,300 adult social care organisations with 40,400 care providing locations and a workforce of around 1.58 million jobs – 78% of which were in the independent sector (private or voluntary organisations) (Skills for Care, 2017).
- According to the health and social care regulator, the Care Quality Commission (2017, p 26):

  In last year's ... report, we said that social care was approaching a tipping point – a point where deterioration in quality would outpace improvement and there would be a significant increase in people whose needs weren't

> being met ... One year on, the overall picture remains precarious, with no long-term solution yet in sight. Demand for care is still increasing through an ageing population with increasingly complex health conditions. At the same time, the capacity of the adult social care sector continues to shrink, with fewer nursing home beds in particular available. Furthermore, more people are having to go without paid care and support at all.

• While 78% of adult social care services are rated as good by the Care Quality Commission and many services have improved on re-inspection, 23% of good services have deteriorated on re-inspection. There are 4,000 fewer nursing home beds since 2015, and 43 councils reported homecare contracts handing back in 2016/17, affecting 3,135 people. Age UK estimate nearly 1.2m older people have unmet care needs.

Social care in an international context

It is harder to find international comparisons of adult social care, but a King's Fund review of nine different countries concluded that 'most countries provide more comprehensive coverage of health care than social care needs, but the gap between the two is generally less stark than in England' (Robertson et al, 2014, p 11). The same review (pp 10–12) found that:

• A number of countries have introduced mandatory insurance to cover social care costs; [but] countries have struggled financially and some have had to cut benefits.
• Most countries surveyed do not have well-functioning private insurance markets to cover social care needs.
• In most countries, accommodation and daily living costs in residential care are not covered by the social insurance programme and make up a large proportion of residents' total bills.
• The family's role in care and the way this is recognised by government differs between countries.

The focus of this book

The *Short Guides* published by Policy Press are designed to provide concise but reliable introductions offering a broad overview of key concepts and topics, and to be accessibly written and jargon-free (but not 'dumbed down' in any way). Key reasons for a *Short Guide to Health and Social Care* are set out below:

- *The topical nature of current debates*: for example, the future of social care funding and the 2017 election; public concerns about current pressures on the NHS; the junior doctors strike and controversial debates about seven-day working; and the previous controversies of the 2012 Lansley reforms – to name but a few.
- *Future careers and study*: people thinking about working in health and social care might want a short introduction to help orientate themselves and decide whether this is an area where they want to pursue a career and/or further study.
- *Overcoming confusion and complexity*: many people are confused by the sheer scale and complexity of health and social care, with lots of jargon, frequent policy changes and new organisations and issues constantly springing up. For all that health and social care are high profile public and political issues, few people understand how the system operates, and many of the key issues remain opaque at best. A good example here is when an international visitor asks you to describe how the health service works. Typically, most people only get a sentence or two in to such a conversation before they realise they don't really know and that their attempts to explain things don't feel very meaningful or convincing. I always come away from such encounters thinking: 'that's a really good question – why do we do it like that?' (and because of my day job, I'm meant to know)!
- *International audiences*: there is significant international interest in the NHS, with a number of international clinicians and managers coming to the UK to learn about the NHS and take key lessons back to their own system.

- *Interagency working*: as explored in Chapters Three and Five, there is an increasing focus on interagency health and social care, with a growing need for material which considers each sector in its own right but also explores the importance/realities/complexity of joint working and common themes across both health and social care.

As set out in Chapter One, social care in England has increasingly become divided into services for adults (overseen by the Department of Health and Social Care) and services for children (overseen by the Department for Education). As a result, this book focuses on health and adult social care, with a separate *Short Guide* by Conradie and Golding (2013) covering work with children and young people. There is also a useful *Short Guide to Social Work* (Adams, 2010), a *Short Guide to Aging and Gerontology* (de Medeiros, 2016) and a broader *Short Guide to Social Policy* (Hudson et al, 2015).

Throughout, the focus is on the UK, albeit including a number of textboxes at intervals to signpost international examples of the same themes in action and to provide further reading. Where a specific piece of legislation or structure is mentioned, this usually refers to the English context, but with references to key differences in other countries of the UK where this illustrates other ways of approaching the same underlying issues. Hopefully this is a helpful way of making the topic manageable, while also demonstrating the breadth and complexity of the issues at stake.

While there are a number of longstanding and successful health and health/social care textbooks (some of which are set out in 'further reading' at the end of this chapter), many of these are more policy orientated and assume a greater level of prior knowledge than the current book. Of the more introductory texts, a number are large edited collections and can be expensive for individual students and new health and social care workers. Because of their size, they can also be difficult to update regularly (despite the very fast-paced nature of recent policy changes). Interestingly, a number of the most popular titles seem to focus on either health or on social care, with few books seeking to provide a short guide for a multidisciplinary audience.

After this introduction, the book is divided into two main sections (with a brief summary and reflections on key messages at the end).

Part 1 contains three chapters focused on '**Structures and services**'. Chapter One provides an overview of the history and structure of current services, looking at how we got to where we are now and setting out a number of themes that run throughout the rest of the book. Chapter Two considers the funding of health and social care, including concepts such as the 'purchaser-provider split', a 'mixed economy of care' and the 'personalisation agenda', as well as the implications of austerity. Chapter Three reviews some of the tensions that exist in the organisation of services – between the local, regional and national; between hospitals and community services; between physical and mental health; between health and social care; and between medical cure and public health/prevention.

Part 2 focuses on '**People and practice**'. Chapter Four looks at the social context in which services operate, exploring concepts such as 'well-being', some of the social factors which contribute to health and the nature of care work. Chapter Five explores 'being a professional', with sections on the nature of professions, values and ethics, power, culture and working with others. Chapter Six moves on to look at delivering care, including a consideration of the relationship between care providers and people receiving care, job satisfaction and stress, and current workforce challenges.

Each chapter tries to summarise the key issues in the main body of the text. Additional material that provides more detailed background or a practical illustration is placed in boxes, tables or diagrams, and categorised in different ways to help readers decide which of these is helpful for them given their particular needs and interests. Early on, there tend to be more 'Facts and Figures' boxes (around the history and structure of services, for example), with greater reference to 'Voices of Experience' later on in the book (where discussion turns to the realities of working in and delivering health and social care).

After each substantive chapter, there is further reading and/or web resources for those who wish to use the chapter as a starting point for following up particular issues in more detail. At the time of going to press, the weblinks in this book were all fully accurate.

However, health and social care websites can change quickly, so some persistence and ingenuity can be required to find such resources further down the line if policy suddenly shifts! Throughout subsequent chapters, key terms are in bold (signalling that these are also explained in the glossary above), as are some of the key sources set out at the end of each chapter.

The following table lists the different types of box to be found in this book, for reference.

Category	Purpose
Facts and Figures	Factual information, key figures and key organisational structures
Voices of Experience	Examples/first-person accounts from professionals, services users and other stakeholders, including NHS or social care national bodies
Key Sources	Extracts from/descriptions of key reports, legislation and guidelines
Concepts and Debates	Explains key ideas, terms and roles (where more detail is needed to explain the main text)

Going back to where this chapter started, this *Short Guide* matters because health and social care matter. As you read this book, it is worth reflecting on (and slightly adapting) a quote from the founder of the NHS, Nye Bevan:

No society can legitimately call itself civilised if a sick person is denied medical aid because of lack of means. (Bevan, 1952, p 100)

To this might be added the contribution of adult social care (which, for reasons set out in Chapter One, has often been a less well understood and more ambiguous service):

No society can legitimately call itself civilised if a sick, frail or disabled person is denied care and support because of lack of means.

Further resources

For people new to health and social care, trade publications such as the *Health Service Journal* or *Community Care* are excellent resources. Whereas the former is available via subscription only, the latter is a free website (www.communitycare.co.uk).

Many **national newspapers** also have sections of their website devoted to the latest health and social care news or to public services more generally (see, for example, www.theguardian.com/society). The BBC news website also has a 'health section' (www.bbc.co.uk/news/health) and (at the time of writing) a section on 'the cost of care' (www.bbc.co.uk/news/health-30782177).

Other books by the same author develop some of the material in this *Short Guide* in greater detail, and may be relevant if readers want to follow up particular themes or to go on to a career or further study in health and social care:

- **Glasby and Dickinson's (2014)** *Partnership Working in Health and Social Care* – as the title suggests, the book is focused on the practicalities of working in joined-up ways across the multitude of agencies that form the health and social care tapestry.
- **Glasby's (2016)** *Understanding Health and Social Care* – this is a good follow-on text to this one, which includes more social policy context and more depth of discussion on particular debates in the health and social care field.

Part 1:

Structures and services

1

History and structure

History matters

Before I trained as a social worker, and later became an academic, I started out as a history student. Perhaps because of this, I've always believed that we need to understand where something has come from to really get a sense of why it is the way it is (and to begin to think through where we might be headed next). This can sometimes be difficult in an era of 24-hour news, social media and new technology, where the emphasis often seems to be on the now and on the future, on rapid/instant dissemination and on the next big thing/trend. In the 2000s, for example, the Labour government branded itself as 'New Labour' and described many of its reforms as a process of 'modernisation'. In many ways, this was an exciting time – but the use of such language (portraying things as dynamic and forward-looking) probably exaggerates the extent to which some things were genuinely 'new'.

Coupled with the pace of current media (and social media), this can contribute to a what often feels a very hyper-active policy context – where political leaders are constantly bombarded with questions and challenges and feel they have respond instantly. This can then exaggerate the sense that something dramatic has happened (it often hasn't), that whatever issue we're facing is the greatest challenge ever, that there's a magic solution which will solve all ills and can be implemented quickly, and that there are clear-cut, easy, soundbite answers.

The result of all this is that we can get lots of strong/heroic claims made in policy documents about what it's possible to achieve; lots of initiatives, pilots and new policies; lots of turnover in political and other leaders; and a corresponding lack of organisational memory. As but one example, I remember being in a meeting where policymakers were keen to set up a 'network' to promote more 'integrated care' (see Chapter Three for further discussion). It fell to me to gently remind them that a previous government had set up an 'Integrated Care Network' (the name/language was identical), that it had been popular and that there had been significant upset when previous policymakers abolished it. This wasn't the fault of anyone present, many of whom were new in role – but it does illustrate how easy it is to lose organisational memory.

To understand current health and social care, we therefore need to understand the past. While Greener (2008) focuses primarily on the NHS, his exploration of 'continuity and change' (the sub-title of his book) identifies a series of '*inheritances*' which help to explain current policy and practice (p 10). I have added 'social care' in brackets to the following quote from his book because the arguments apply equally across both arenas:

- To understand the problems of the NHS [and social care] reform today, it is necessary to understand earlier organisational forms and the inheritances they bring to policy today.
- Policy makers inherit health [and social] services that are the result of previous decisions and are underpinned by ideas and structures that the present government may find outdated or even wholly objectionable. It is by explaining how they deal with these inheritances that health reform can be explored from a new perspective, explaining why some reforms work and others do not.
- Understanding the NHS [and social care] in terms of a series of inheritances is useful because it forces an explanation of exactly how they come to limit the choices of policy makers and those working in health [and social] services.

Where have we come from?

In 1948, a leaflet was sent to every household in the country, introducing the new NHS (reproduced online by the Socialist Health Association – www.sochealth.co.uk/national-health-service/the-sma-and-the-foundation-of-the-national-health-service-dr-leslie-hilliard-1980/the-start-of-the-nhs-1948/).

> Your new National Health Service begins on 5th July … It will provide you with all medical, dental and nursing care. Everyone – rich or poor, man, woman of child – can use it or any part of it. There are no charges, except for a few special items. But it is not a "charity". You are all paying for it, mainly as taxpayers, and it will relieve your money worries in times of illness.

2018 was therefore the 70th anniversary of the NHS (as well as of the passage of the **National Assistance Act**, often seen as the founding legislation for the current adult social care system). As the NHS Choices website explains:

> Since its launch in 1948, the NHS has grown to become the world's largest publicly funded health service. It is also one of the most efficient, most egalitarian and most comprehensive. The NHS was born out of a long-held ideal that good healthcare should be available to all, regardless of wealth – a principle that remains at its core. (www.nhs.uk/nhsengland/thenhs/nhshistory/pages/the-nhs%20history.aspx)

This must have felt revolutionary (see the Summary at the end of this book for some real-life examples). However, the birth of the NHS was as much the result of a gradual evolution as it was an overnight revolution, with a number of key developments over time (see **Facts and Figures 2**). While the creation of the post-war adult social care system was probably less dramatic and more embryonic, the end of the notorious **Poor Law** was a cause for celebration. When I trained as a social worker, I met older people who remembered what life was like before the welfare state, and who still associated going into a care home with 'going to the workhouse'. For all the imperfections of current adult social care, these older people were incredibly grateful for what little we could provide, and their experience of services (which I didn't think were good enough) contrasted sharply with the experiences which their parents might have had just a generation previously.

Interestingly, many of the key changes in **Facts and Figures 2** seem to have come during periods of severe crisis and upheaval (for example, the rapid urbanisation and industrialisation of the 19th century, coupled with conflicts such as the Crimean and Boer Wars; the First and Second World Wars; the Wall Street Crash/ Great Depression; and – later on in this chapter – the international economic crises of the 1970s). Although this is a significant over-simplification, there is probably an important lesson here. While politicians often claim to be introducing radical reforms (and while policies might look significantly different at face value), it can often be difficult to bring about fundamental change unless there is some sort of major crisis which forces us as a society to question the status quo. This is not to say that we are powerless to improve things outside such periods of crisis – but it often feels that what is possible at any given time is constrained by strong political, social, economic and cultural forces, with only occasional windows when something fundamentally new becomes temporarily possible.

Facts and Figures 2: A very brief history of health and social care

19th century and before	• The medical profession has evolved since Medieval and Tudor Times, with 'physicians', 'barber-surgeons' and 'apothecaries' evolving into doctors focused on diagnosis and medical treatment ('medics'), surgeons and general practitioners (GPs). • For those unable to work or to support themselves, the main source of 'support' was the **Poor Law**, with workhouses made as harsh as possible to deter all but the most needy. • Doctors were private practitioners charging a fee for their service. • Over time, there emerged a mix of voluntary and municipal (local government) hospitals with no overall coordination.
Late 19th century	• During the late 19th century/early 20th century, there were a series of reforms designed to improve public health and services for women and children (sometimes in response to periods of warfare and concerns about the physical condition of future troops). • Public anxiety about extreme poverty in Britain's big cities led to a series of voluntary organisations providing welfare services at local or national level. • Modern social work has its origins in the Charity Organisation Society (COS), which sought to coordinate the provision of charity and assessed individuals to see who was deserving of assistance.
Early–mid-20th century	• During the 20th century, there was a gradual extension of access to health care (funded via National Insurance), but often only for people in work. Pensions and sickness/unemployment payments also began to be paid to some groups. • During the Second World War, the **Emergency Medical Service** provided a more planned, comprehensive system, while the experience of war led to greater government intervention in various aspects of life. As its name implies, the focus was understandably on preparing for mass casualties, on hospital services and on medical cure. • The 1942 **Beveridge Report** set out a vision for what has become known as the post-war welfare state. After the war, there was widespread optimism and a desire to create a better society for the future (as well as a socialist government committed to greater state provision of welfare, funded by general taxation).

Mid-20th century	• In 1946, the **National Health Service Act** created the NHS (implemented in 1948), with care provided free at the point of delivery. While some government Ministers wanted to create a system based within local government, the Minister for Health and Housing (Aneurin Bevan) wanted to create a national system, taking previous voluntary and municipal hospitals into national ownership. This ultimately led to a compromise, whereby hospitals became part of a national system, community health and social services were provided by local government, and GPs remained as independent contractors - an approach known as the 'tri-partite system'. • In 1948, the **National Assistance Act** replaced the Poor Law with a national system of financial payments to those in needs (social security) and services run by local councils to provide practical support to older and disabled people (social care). • During many of these changes, the medical profession was hostile to an extension of government control over its work, and the British Medical Association led fierce resistance to the idea of a National Health Service. This led to a series of compromises, with GPs remaining as private practitioners selling their services to the government, hospital doctors retaining the right to engage in private practice, doctors having significant influence at many levels of the new service and a generous system of merit payments for senior doctors. Reflecting on this, Bevan described how he had 'stuffed their [doctors'] mouths with gold'.

As a result of these inheritances and compromises, there are a number of features of current services which make more sense when seen in historical perspective (see **Facts and Figures 3**).

Facts and Figures 3: Key features of health and social care

Key features	Why they matter
A commitment to funding health care for all from general taxation, with services based on clinical need rather than on people's ability to pay	This means that the NHS has strong egalitarian principles (it tries to treat everyone the same and sees fairness and equality as really important). These are key values, but can also lead to complexities. For example: • Chapter Two explores the funding of health and social care, recognising that, if services are universal and free, then there has to be a way to manage demand (for example, people may need to wait for services rather than being able to pay to access care instantly). • Chapter Four discusses whether 'treating everyone the same' is the best way to achieve these laudable aims, or whether we sometimes have to treat some people differently in order to achieve similar outcomes for different groups of people in different circumstances.
A separate system of health (NHS) and social care (local government) services	Creates difficulties working across boundaries where people have complex or multiple needs.
A tripartite system, with different roles for hospitals, community health services and general practice	Practical and cultural barriers emerge between: • Hospital services (a national, better funded, more prestigious system); • Community health services (initially run by local government and often under-funded and low status – so-called 'Cinderella services'); • General practice (independent contractors).
A significant division between cash for people in need (social security) and practical support for disabled or frail people (social care)	Separate systems emerge for social security and for social care, despite the fact that many people may access both systems, and that the focus of each service may overlap.

A very powerful position for doctors	Tensions between the autonomy of the medical profession and the role of the state in funding/providing a national system. This is sometimes described as the **double-bed relationship** (the state needs doctors to deliver health care, and doctors have to work with the state given it is the main funder of health care). Patients have often had a passive role, with an assumption that 'doctor knows best'.
A tendency to focus on buildings-based services (hospitals and former workhouses) and on meeting the needs of people with severe needs/in crisis	Less emphasis on services in the community, in people's own homes and on prevention.
A tendency to focus on physical health problems	A relative neglect of the needs of people with mental health problems or learning disabilities.
A focus on medical cure	Less emphasis on supporting people with chronic (ongoing) diseases.

Since the foundation of the NHS and the passage of the **National Assistance Act** in 1948, both health and social services have continued to evolve. Although more detailed policy overviews are available in some of the further reading recommended at the end of this chapter, key changes/themes are set out in **Facts and Figures 4**.

The current health and social care system is described in more detail in **Facts and Figures 5**. As an example of the sheer complexity of these structures, **Facts and Figures 6** depicts a 'simplified' version of the English system from 2017 – which would be utterly incomprehensible to anyone without very specialist knowledge, and gives an insight into just how difficult any form of joint working across organisational boundaries is likely to be.

Facts and Figures 4: Recent history of health and social care

1940s onwards	Initial optimism that providing universal health care would reduce costs over time, as the health of the population increased. In practice, the new NHS faced an immediate backlog of ill health. It was also able to restore people to health, only for them to become ill again in future – thus increasing rather than decreasing costs. As the population has aged and technology has advanced, we have achieved significant increases in life expectancy but also in costs (with services effectively the victim of their own success). Over time, the NHS has seemed to need a long-term average annual increase in funding of around 4% in order to keep up with rising needs and demands, and any less than this over time means significant funding and service pressures. However, these are political choices in a tax-funded system – the government of the day decides how much money to provide, and services have to try to deliver the best care possible with what they have at any given time.
1950s	Because of initial and ongoing financial challenges, charges were introduced for items such as prescriptions and dentistry in the early 1950s, contributing to Bevan's resignation.
1960s	Increased reaction against the provision of care to people with mental health problems, learning disabilities or dementia in long-stay hospitals, fuelled in part by a series of abuse scandals. Over time, there has been growing recognition that many services can be provided in the community, and that these groups deserve the same choices and control over their lives as anyone else. Seebohm report led to the creation of more generic social services departments (working with both children and adults). Prior to this, social care had been fragmented between work with children, welfare services for older people, mental health, social work, and other specialisms.
1970s	From 1974, the NHS was reorganised in order to create a more unified system, with community health services and public health transferring out of local government. While this created more unified NHS services, it could also be seen as creating more fragmented health and social care. The development of Community Health Councils was an attempt to introduce a lay voice into debates about the health service, seeking the involvement of local people in improving care. These were later abolished and have been replaced with a series of different mechanisms for public and patient engagement in the NHS – many of which have been short-lived, under-funded and/or lacking in impact.

1980s	Following the economic crises of the 1970s and the subsequent election of Margaret Thatcher, Conservative governments in the 1980s and early 1990s sought to introduce greater competition in health and social care. The NHS **internal market** (or **purchaser–provider split**) created a situation where (in England) Health Authorities (now **Clinical Commissioning Groups**) decide what care is needed on behalf of a local area, and fund this from a range of different providers (who compete with each other to secure this 'business'). This is meant to improve quality and 'customer service' but has also led to criticisms that competition is not a good way to organise health services and that care is being privatised (see Chapter Two). As part of these changes, a review of the NHS argued for the introduction of **general management**, incorporating a number of tools and techniques from the private sector into public services.
1990s	In social care, the **community care reforms** built on similar logic, turning social workers into 'care managers' who would assess need and purchase the care that was needed for individuals from a mix of public, private and voluntary providers. Over time, the bulk of services became provided by the private sector – and there were significant problems in the 2010s when a number of very large care homes providers (owning tens of thousands of beds) encountered significant financial problems (raising the risk that such a company might go bust, leaving many thousands of frail older people at risk). There were also high profile abuse scandals and broader concerns about the quality and appropriateness of care provided in some private sector assessment and treatment centres for people with profound learning disabilities and challenging behaviour.
2000s	In the 2000s, there was significant and sustained investment in health and social care from the New Labour government. In return for extra funding, services were expected to become much more responsive to the needs of patients/service users and to meet a series of challenging service standards (for example, around waiting times in A&E). With extra money and significant policy focus, access to services improved significantly and waiting times declined dramatically.

2010s

Over time, there have been repeated reorganisations of the NHS – often conducted in the name of reforming services but probably serving more to disrupt existing care, causing a distraction for staff and managers, and reducing morale and productivity in the short term. This has been criticised by a range of commentators as providing a veneer of change, but actually making things worse rather than better – but this tendency to look to structural changes as an apparent 'solution' shows no sign of abating. Despite pledging no more top-down reorganisations, the Lansley reforms (described later in this box) were described by the then NHS chief executive as 'so big you can see them from space'.

Also in the 2010s, social services departments in England were broken up into services for children and services for adults (following a high profile child death). Some areas have since appointed a single person to head up both directorates, or have sought to maintain separate children's/education services by putting adult social care together with housing, communities or leisure.

From 2010, the Coalition government pursued a policy of austerity and reductions in public spending. Although the NHS budget was protected, it has failed to increase at the pace of need and demand, and local government budgets have experienced drastic cuts. Services have therefore been under sustained pressure for a number of years, with significant financial deficits, with widespread public, professional, medical and political anxieties about what the future may hold and about the extent to which the current Conservative government was sufficiently sighted on the scale of the issues. In England, controversial health reforms introduced by Andrew Lansley in 2012 created a very fragmented system, with a series of different national bodies responsible for different parts of the system and a lack of local or regional leadership to help respond to the substantial challenges we face. Local **Health and Wellbeing Boards** (formed jointly between the NHS and local government) are one way of trying to join this fragmented system back up and to promote further joint working.

As part of the Lansley reforms, the lead responsibility for public health transferred to local government (where it had been based prior to 1974). However, widespread cuts to local government budgets have decimated public health programmes in many parts of England.

In adult social care, the funding of long-term care for older people has been an underlying and controversial issue for more than two decades, with a number of different attempts to review the system subsequently failing to be implemented and/or being kicked into the long grass. At the time of writing, the signs are that this might be happening again, with no government seeming willing to grasp this difficult issue and pursue a coherent, long-term solution.

Facts and Figures 5: Health and social care across the UK

Health and social care have been more formally integrated since the early 1970s.

At the time of writing, a single Health and Social Care Board commissions services from six Health and Social Care Trusts (five of which provide integrated health and social care services; the sixth provides ambulance services).

In Scotland, 14 NHS Boards deliver local health services (with a number of Scotland-wide Special Boards responsible for things such as public health, ambulance services and education/training). The previous purchaser-provider split was abolished in 2004 (unified NHS Boards now decide what services are needed and provide these at local level, rather than having separate Trusts to provide services commissioned by Boards). Adult social care is the responsibility of Social Work Departments within 32 local councils. The Public Bodies (Joint Working) (Scotland) Act 2014, brings together health and social care services through 31 local partnerships, managing around £8 billion.

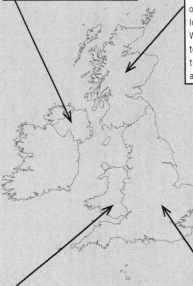

In England, Clinical Commissioning Groups decide what health services are needed locally and fund these from NHS Trusts, as well as from private/voluntary sector organisations. More specialist services are commissioned nationally by NHS England. Adult social care is part of local councils (sometimes a Directorate in its own right, sometimes integrated with children's services or sometimes working alongside services such as housing or leisure). Social care commissioners purchase services from a range of public, private and voluntary sector providers, with most care delivered in the independent sector. Health and Wellbeing Boards assess the needs of the local area and agree a joint strategy to promote health and well-being.

In Wales, a 2009 reorganisation ended the purchaser–provider split, replacing 22 Local Health Boards and 7 NHS Trusts with 7 unified Local Health Boards.

These plan and deliver healthcare in their areas, with three national Trusts focusing on public health, cancer care and ambulance services.

Social services are delivered by 22 local councils.

Facts and Figures 6: The Structure of Health and Social Care in England

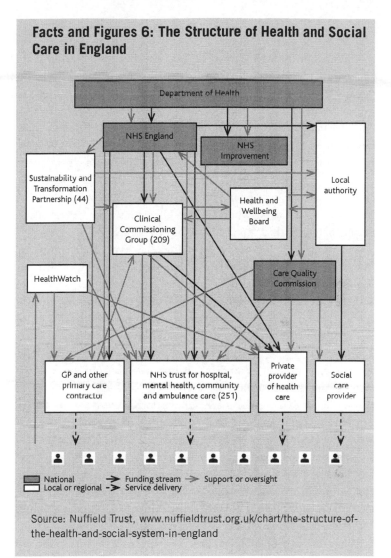

Source: Nuffield Trust, www.nuffieldtrust.org.uk/chart/the-structure-of-the-health-and-social-system-in-england

Unfortunately, most accounts of UK services focus on developments in England, without recognising that the health and social care systems that have developed in the four countries of the UK are very different (particularly since the devolution of greater powers to Wales, Scotland and Northern Ireland in the late 1990s/early 2000s). This means that there is considerable scope for us to learn from developments across other parts of the UK, creating scope for what might be seen as a 'natural experiment'. However, it has sometimes felt as if the politics of devolution have stopped us from doing this as much as might have been the case, with a greater willingness for England to look to somewhere like the US or Australia/New Zealand rather than to Wales, Scotland and Northern Ireland.

Internationally, the UK system that has evolved over time is unusual in a number of respects (see **Facts and Figures 7**). While it is important that we look for good practice examples from elsewhere and seek to learn from these wherever it gives scope to improve services, there are also risks inherent in trying to import ways of working from other systems which seem to work in that particular context, but which might not translate to a different system. Often, such practice examples can teach us important lessons for our own system, and give us a more objective, critical lens with which to re-look at our own services ('why do we do X like that?') – but there are seldom 'magic answers' that another system has solved and that we could import wholesale. Some people find this dispiriting (on one level, it would be great if there was an easy answer somewhere else that we had simply overlooked). However, others find it reassuring (other people are also struggling with some of the things that we find hard – and this might be because they are genuinely difficult: if they were easy, we would have solved them by now!).

When comparing the welfare systems in different countries, commentators often draw on a framework first developed by Esping-Anderson (1990), which distinguishes between different welfare 'regimes' (see **Concepts and Debates 1**).

Concepts and Debates 1: Different welfare regimes

Welfare regime	Example	Key features
Social Democratic	Sweden	Committed to full employment and generous welfare provision
Corporatist/ Conservative	Germany	Well-developed services with a mix of private contributions and social insurance
Liberal	US	Limited public welfare and a key role for families, charities and religious organisations

Source: Esping-Andersen (1990)

Facts and Figures 7: The UK system in an international context

Using the Esping-Andersen approach outlined above, the UK seems something of a hybrid, with a mix of elements over time. In health and social care, unusual features of our system include (www.kingsfund.org.uk/blog/2014/03/what-can-we-learn-how-other-countries-fund-health-and-social-care) the following:

- Our NHS is the largest publicly funded health service in the world, and many of its services are free at the point of delivery. It is one of the leading systems worldwide in terms of safety, access, equity and administrative efficiency.
- Our adult social care services are often more separated from social security (cash payments to those in need) than in some other countries.
- The division between the organisation and funding of our health and social services is more pronounced than in some systems.
- Family and friends caring for others face a number of challenges, but UK carers were the first internationally to have access to tax concessions (1967), to a state welfare benefit (1976), to a social care assessment of their needs (1995) and to the right to request flexible working (2002) (www.ippr.org/juncture/caring-for-our-carers).

Looking at expenditure on health care as a proportion of **GDP** (a measure of a country's economy), the UK spends less than near neighbours such as France, Germany and the Netherlands, less than most Scandinavian countries, less than Canada and Japan, and much less than the US (the highest spender). Of the G7 countries (a group of countries with large developed economies), the UK spent the second lowest proportion of **GDP** (only Italy spent less).

Looking back at the history of UK services (as well as other systems internationally), it is clear that there is no perfect way of organising a health and social care system. Often, the same debates have re-occurred over time, and our current services are the product of gradual evolution, a series of trade-offs and a number of pragmatic decisions about how best to respond to the challenges of the day. While a new policymaker may want to pursue a radical agenda or introduce a sudden change, there are usually a series of practical and political constraints as to what is feasible at any given moment in time, and so what happens in practice is often closer to what happened before than was originally intended. As a result, there are a series of ongoing themes in policy debates which recur throughout this book (and which are discussed in greater detail in later chapters).

Concepts and Debates 2: Key policy debates and themes

A tendency to introduce significant structural reorganisations as a way of trying to improve services (despite the reality that this often proves a distraction for managers and staff, can make some things worse, and only gives a false impression of change)

Ongoing debates about how best to fund health and social care, with a sense that however much is currently available is never enough, frequent discussions about the impact of changing demography and society, and a repeated failure to 'grasp the nettle' of the funding of long-term care

Ongoing tensions between the local, regional and national

Which services should be provided in hospital and which could be delivered in the community

How to meet physical and mental health needs

How to treat people who are seriously ill or injured, while also preventing ill health and promoting independence

How best to join up health and social care in a system not designed with joint work in mind

The different perspectives of patients, doctors and managers, and the interplay of these over time

How best to manage and lead services that depend on the technical skills of professionals who may be experts in their individual fields, but that need to be organised in a way which can cope with significant complexity, volume and pace, and make best use of scarce resources

How best to support people to deliver high quality, compassionate care and to deal with the incredible emotional stresses that working in health and social care can entail

Similarly, Powell's (2018) review of anniversary documents (comparing key official documents for each decade of the NHS) suggests that pressures first identified in the 1950s – ageing populations, the cost of technological advances and rising public expectations – have been with us throughout (see also Timmins, 2008). Despite periods of continuity and of change, policymakers over time have often looked to similar solutions:

> [F]or many years reports have stressed the visions such as integrated, seamless and more person-centred care; more care delivered in primary and community settings; and a greater focus

on prevention. Moreover, many of these visions are common
to other health care systems. (Powell, 2018, p 5)

As the health and social care system celebrated its 70th anniversary
in 2018, no doubt similar challenges and potential solutions will
continue to be debated going forwards.

Different political ideologies and cultures

One of the ways of trying to understand how our services have
changed over time is to think about the political beliefs and goals of
different governments (as well as the broader cultural assumptions
common at any given moment in time). In the UK, political parties
are often characterised as 'left' or 'right-wing':

- *Left-wing governments* tend to emphasise the importance of a strong
  state to meet the needs of citizens, the public ownership of such
  services and higher taxes to pay for such provision.
- *Right-wing governments* tend to stress the importance of low taxes
  (so that people have an incentive to work hard and to look after
  themselves and their families) and the role of the market in helping
  people choose what services they want.
- Over time, a number of different parties have tried to occupy *the
  centre ground* between these two extremes, portraying themselves as
  appealing to the 'average person on the street' or the 'floating' or
  'swing voter' (who does not have strong party political affiliations).

In UK elections, the electoral system in based on a 'first past the post'
system, where the candidate with the largest votes becomes the local
Member of Parliament (MP), and where the party with the largest
number of MPs is usually able to form a government (typically the
Conservatives or Labour as the two largest parties). This is different to
various countries in continental Europe, where there can be a strong
traditional of proportional representation (whereby the number of
seats depends on the percentage of the vote won, not on winning
an outright majority at local level), with a tendency for a series of

smaller parties to come together to form a Coalition government. At times when the major UK parties fundamentally disagree with each other on ideological grounds, our system means that there can be sudden shifts in policy when a new government is elected (as with the election of Margaret Thatcher in 1979, for example). Equally, when the parties are relatively close together in terms of underlying ideology and competing for the centre ground, there can be a focus on a relatively small number of constituencies where the local seat is genuinely up for grabs (but perhaps a corresponding neglect of areas that are overwhelmingly likely to vote for a particular party and unlikely to change allegiances). For those in the health and social care sector trying to make sense of all this, there is therefore a risk of sudden lurches in policy and priorities, or a political reluctance to tackle underlying issues that might alienate swing voters. Understanding the politics of the day can therefore be important for people working in and leading services.

At a broader level, the implications of different political ideologies (and difficult cultural contexts) can also be seen by looking at different health and social care systems internationally. In the US, for example, critics of Barack Obama's health reforms have argued that the ability to choose who provides your health care is a fundamental right, and that government has no place in intervening in something as fundamental as people's health (criticising this for being a form of 'socialised medicine'). Rather than increasing tax to provide better services, the emphasis has often been on tax cuts (to give people a greater incentive to be entrepreneurial, hard-working and innovative). This is very different to Scandinavian countries, where there is a strong tradition of the state playing a key role in meeting the welfare needs of its citizens, with people more content to contribute taxes to a strong state. In some Mediterranean, African and Asian countries, there has traditionally been a stronger emphasis on family and local community, with fewer formal services and a greater cultural expectation that families (often women) will 'look after their own'. This might be less acceptable in a society with a strong commitment to tackling gender inequality and to greater female participation in the labour market (and indeed is often perceived as breaking down in countries where rapid social changes are leading to families being more geographically dispersed and less able to care for each other). Whether you see each of these different approaches as 'right' or 'wrong' can often depend on personal and political beliefs, but these are also heavily influenced by the kind of society in which we have grown up. Thus, what is 'normal' often depends on the eye of the beholder (see Chapter Four for further discussion of **social construction**).

Further resources

NHS England provides an online introduction to the NHS, with a helpful film/animation about how the NHS works and links to various organisational charts explaining how the NHS is structured and how money flows (www.england.nhs.uk/participation/nhs/).

The **NHS Choices** website explains:

- the history of the NHS (www.nhs.uk/NHSEngland/thenhs/ nhshistory/pages/the-nhs history.aspx)
- how the NHS is organised and key features of its structure (www. nhs.uk/NHSEngland/thenhs/about/Pages/nhsstructure.aspx)

Elsewhere in the UK:

- The **Scottish Parliament Information Centre** (SPICe) has produced an introduction to the NHS in Scotland (www. parliament.scot/ResearchBriefingsAndFactsheets/S5/SB_16-100_The_National_Health_Service_in_Scotland.pdf).
- **NHS Wales** summarises the structure of the Welsh NHS (www. wales.nhs.uk/nhswalesaboutus/structure).
- **Northern Ireland's Health and Social Care Online** sets out the Northern Ireland system (in which health and social care are integrated), with links to key local and national bodies (http:// online.hscni.net/home/hsc-structure/).

Helpful **anniversary reviews** of the NHS are provided (at 60) by Timmins (2008) and (at 70) by Powell (2018).

In terms of **adult social care**:

- The King's Fund provides a series of short videos to explain 'what is social care and how does it work?' (including how it is funded and how it works with other services; see www.kingsfund.org. uk/projects/what-is-social-care).
- The House of Commons Library has produced a helpful briefing on adult social care in England (including what it is, who provides it, how it is paid for, pressures on services and long-term sustainability; http://researchbriefings.parliament.uk/ResearchBriefing/Summary/CBP-7903).
- In Scotland, the Social Work Services Strategic Forum has published a vision for adult social care, with key statistics and an overview of priorities (www.gov.scot/Resource/0047/00473374. pdf).
- The Welsh government provides information on the implications of the Social Services and Wellbeing (Wales) Act 2014 (http://gov. wales/topics/health/socialcare/act/?skip=1&lang=en).
- In Northern Ireland, services are more formally integrated (see http://online.hscni.net/home/hsc-structure/).

Helpful **textbooks** which contain summaries of the history of health and/or social care and more recent reforms/debates include:

- Baggott's (2011) *Public Health Policy and Politics* and (2013) *Partnerships for Public Health and Well-being* – these are detailed but accessible summaries of the key issues in public health (often a neglected topic);
- Glasby's (2016) *Understanding Health and Social Care* – see 'Further resources' at the end of the Introduction for a brief description;
- Greener's (2008) *Healthcare in the UK* – history of the NHS, showing how services are influenced by historical legacies and the broader social/political context (also includes a specific chapter

on nursing, which is a profession often neglected in key NHS textbooks);

- Ham's (2009) *Health Policy in Britain* – a classic textbook from a leading commentator;
- Hunter's (2016) *The Health Debate* – analysis and personal assessment of key policy tensions;
- Klein's (2013) *The New Politics of the NHS* – key and very readable analysis of the policy changes that have shaped our current health services;
- Means et al's (2008) *Community Care* – particularly strong on social care services for older people, and great at helping to make sense of key issues by putting current issues in a historical context.

For different **political ideologies** and the impact of these on public services, Alcock et al's (2016) *Student's Guide to Social Policy* contains bite-sized chapters in a short section on 'Key perspectives'.

Looking across the different systems of the UK, key comparisons include:

- Analysis of the performance of the four health systems of the UK commissioned by The Health Foundation and the Nuffield Trust (Bevan et al, 2014);
- Lessons for England from integrated care in Northern Ireland, Scotland and Wales (Ham et al, 2013);
- Analysis of **free personal care** in Scotland to inform English debates around funding options (Dickinson et al, 2007);
- Reflections on social care's experience of joint working in the four countries of the UK (ADASS et al, 2014);
- Heenan and Birrell's (2018) analysis of integrated care in the four countries of the UK.

2

Funding health and social care

As this chapter was being written, both health and social care were facing massive and unprecedented financial challenges. While the NHS was facing what is believed to be the longest period of sustained disinvestment in its history, adult social care was reeling after many years of stringent local government cuts (described by one council leader as 'the end of local government as we know it'). These are important and emotive issues, with much at stake, as the newspaper coverage in **Voices of Experience 2** illustrates. Of course, this is one newspaper, with its own editorial stance on the issues at stake, and the different quotes show how a range of different issues can quickly become rolled up in a discussion about funding.

To place these debates in a broader context, this chapter explores:

- different approaches to funding health and social care;
- the **purchaser–provider split** in both health and social care and the implications of **commissioning**;
- the reality and implications of a **mixed economy of care**;
- the impact of austerity;
- controversies surrounding the funding of long-term care; and
- the **personalisation** agenda.

Voices of Experience 2: NHS funding in the headlines

Thousands of people joined a demonstration in London ending at Downing Street on Saturday in protest at what they say is the crisis facing the NHS.

Marchers were addressed by speakers who outlined their experience of the pressures facing the NHS. One mother told how her daughter died after she had been allowed out of psychiatric care too soon.

Nicky Romero sobbed as she told of the death of her daughter, Becky. 'What kind of future will our children have if they can't get the help they need?' her mother asked. 'If the NHS was properly funded my daughter might still be alive.'

Source: NHS Protest: thousands march to demand more cash for NHS, *Guardian*, 4 February 2018, www.theguardian.com/uk-news/2018/feb/04/nhs-budget-cuts-march-protest-jeremy-hunt-london-funding

The NHS is funded primarily through general taxation (including National Insurance contributions), with patient fees and charges for prescriptions or dentistry accounting for just over 1% of the NHS budget in 2015–16 (see King's Fund, 2017, for all statistics in this paragraph). Across the UK, just over 10% of the population have a private health insurance policy (usually offered by employers as part of people's overall package). While countries such as Canada, Australia, New Zealand and the Scandinavian countries also rely heavily on tax funding, they include greater levels of funding from user charges or insurance. Canada, for example, funds about 70% of health spending through public means.

As we saw in Chapter One, this way of funding the NHS means that:

1. Care is typically provided free at the point of delivery, based on clinical need rather than people's ability to pay. This provides an inspiring vision, and ensures much more equal access to health care than in countries where the poor are deterred from seeking help by high out-of-pocket costs or the cost of insurance premiums.

2. We all have a vested interest in the NHS (as patients, taxpayers and voters) and health care is a crucial topic for the media and politicians. While the NHS enjoys lots of public and political support, and tends to have its budget protected relative to other services, it also means that politicians feel they need to be seen to be intervening in the health service if they are to retain the support of voters. Although politicians would say that they need to have a say if the public holds them to account for how the health service does, many people working in the NHS would say that politicians intervene too much in the day-to-day running of the service, and that this is unhelpful.

3. It is ultimately a political decision as to how much money the NHS receives, and NHS leaders needs to work out how best to use the funding they are allocated to make it work as best it can. However much we gave the NHS it could always spend more if more was available, so it has to make some hard choices about how to spend the money it has got. Equally, a service of this scale could always find way of spending some of its money better, no matter how efficient it is, so the need to deliver appropriate savings to reinvest elsewhere is a constant challenge.

4. With a finite budget, and providing care free on the basis of need, there has to be a way to manage demand. This basically means that we often have to wait for care, both because other more urgent cases may come in, and because there has to be a way of rationing access. In the late 1990s, after a significant period of underfunding, some waiting times were very long indeed, and people could wait over two years for a number of hospital services. After a dramatic and prolonged increase in NHS funding under New Labour (1997–2010), waits came down and most people were seen within A&E within 4 hours and within 18 weeks from

referral to treatment (still a long time but a remarkable reduction). Since 2010, service and funding pressures have been growing, and it is proving impossible to hold on to these achievements. NHS leaders are currently engaged in a brave discussion with government and the public, trying to be very clear that we either need to pay more if we want to hit these targets, or we need to expect less – but that we cannot continue to deliver such waiting times on the current basis.

5. In addition to managing demand via waiting lists, the NHS has a series of mechanisms for deciding what kind of care is appropriate to fund. At local level (in England), **CCGs** decide what services are needed on behalf of the local population, and secure these from a range of different providers (see the discussion of **commissioning** and a **mixed economy of care** later in this chapter). If there are very specific reasons why an individual or a small group of people may need something different, then there is a local process to make individual funding requests. At a national level, NHS England funds the provision of specialist services, while the National Institute for Health and Care Excellence (NICE) makes evidence-based recommendations on effective, good value health care (including well-established methodologies for judging the effectiveness and cost effectiveness of new medicines and technologies; see www.nice.org.uk).

Adult social care is funded in a very different way to the NHS, via a mix of central government grants allocated to local councils, local taxation and a significant role for user charges. These can be politically unpopular, and charging for adult social care is an increasingly hot topic nationally (this is discussed further later in this chapter). With health care free at the point of delivery and adult social care subject to charges, it can make a huge difference to the individual as to whether their needs are seen as the responsibility of the NHS or of local councils – especially if these needs fall in the grey area between health and social care.

Having planned how much money they are likely to receive from different sources, councils can then choose how they set their budgets, and may wish to prioritise particular services or functions depending on local needs and context. This is important, as it means that central government does not give councils a set amount of money to spend on adult social care. Instead, councils receive some money centrally for the range of different functions they provide, raise money through local taxes and user charges, and then decide what to spend on adult social care. In practice, significant cuts in local government funding mean that all budgets are under massive pressure. While many councils have tried to protect their children's and adult social care services as much as possible (with other services being cut even further), they are effectively 'caught between a rock and a hard place', with rising need and significant financial challenges creating a real sense of crisis at the frontline. This was described by one council leader as 'the end of local government as we know it' (the austerity agenda is discussed later in this chapter).

This method of funding adult social care is important for two reasons:

1. Historically there has been a balance between central and local funding (although this is changing in an era of austerity with dramatic reductions in central funding). This means that local people contribute towards the cost of local services via user charges and local taxes, but that there is a national mechanism for a degree of redistribution. If we only funded our social and other services locally, then poor areas (which might have high levels of need) would end up paying the most (this is referred to as 'regressive'). Instead, the central element of local government funding ensures that there is an attempt to balance out this aspect of the budget, using a complex formula that tries to take account of the extent of local needs. For example, some services will cost more in an area with lots of older people, some services will be more expensive if there are lots of children, some needs might be greater in poorer areas, and some services might be more expensive to provide in very sparsely populated rural areas.

2. If central funds are fixed (or if they reduce), any local spending pressure has to fall on local taxes and user charges. Not only are

there strict rules governing how much councils can increase local taxes by, but this also tends to be very unpopular, and too high a rise can lead to the council being voted out at the next elections. This process is very clever and is entirely deliberate, as a way of keeping local spending down. By way of illustration (using made-up numbers to keep it simple):

- Let's say that a council had a budget of £100 (made up of £80 from central sources and £20 from local tax/charges).
- If it wanted to increase its spending to £105 to meet more need or provide better services, it would only be increasing its overall spending by £5 (5%).
- However, all of this increase would need to be funded by the local portion of the budget, which would rise from £20 to £25 (an increase of 25%).
- Thus, a 5% increase in overall spending has led to a 25% increase in local tax/charges – and is likely to be incredibly locally unpopular, thus putting the council under pressure not to make this fairly modest increase.

This is known as the **gearing** effect, and means that councils have typically been under significant pressure to constrain spending (even in times of generous funding). In one sense, some of these dilemmas are reducing in England as central funding is dramatically cut, and more and more pressure is falling on local taxes/charges anyway. However, as demand has grown over time, central government has also placed limits on the amount by which local government can increase local council tax each year (known as **capping**). These limits have typically been very tight, although it is a measure of the pressure on social care that councils are now being allowed to increase tax by more, specifically to fund adult social care. Many regard these council tax increases as unsustainable or a 'sticking plaster' solution. Certainly, they cannot go on unchecked without further political difficulty and seem a poor substitute for a more fundamental rethink on how society funds social care.

In terms of what care is then provided, councils set out eligibility criteria, describing what level of need they will meet. These local

criteria were later combined into a national framework (known as
'Fair Access to Care Services' or FACS). Under the **Care Act 2014**,
there is a national minimum threshold for adult care and support
(see www.scie.org.uk/care-act-2014/assessment-and-eligibility/
eligibility/definition.asp for further details).

Commissioning and the purchaser–provider split

In the 1990s, the Conservative governments (in power from 1979
to 1997) introduced a series of changes to health and social care,
trying to make the sector more 'business-like' and to learn lessons
from private enterprise. They believed that people were paying too
much of their income in taxes, to fund public services that were
too large and inefficient, and that this took away people's need to
be responsible for themselves and their families. By leaving more
money in people's own hands, it was believed that innovative and
entrepreneurial people would be able to set up new businesses,
generate more wealth and employ more people, with the spending of
these wealthy individuals 'trickling down' and benefitting everyone.

In the NHS, this led to the introduction of general managers,
who would bring new skills from outside the health service and
introduce more innovative private sector techniques. There was
also a new **purchaser–provider split**, with organisations (initially
known as Health Authorities, later Primary Care Trusts and now
CCGs) responsible for deciding what services an area needed and
funding these from a range of different providers (who could be
from the public, private or voluntary sector). Hospital, community
health, mental health and ambulance services were provided by
NHS Trusts, who were public bodies but with Boards modelled
on those common in the private sector (including a number of
Non-Executive Directors, who might well be from outside the
NHS from backgrounds in business, law or finance). Bodies such
as Health Authorities would thus sign annual contracts with their
local Trusts, setting out a certain amount of care to be provided for
a certain price. This was meant to give a greater incentive to Trusts
to be more innovative and efficient. Over time, a national system

of payments was introduced (**Payment by Results**) and patients were able to choose which hospital they wanted to receive their care from, with greater information available about the nature and quality of care delivered (a policy known as **Patient Choice**). This was meant to make NHS Trusts compete with each other to attract people's 'business' or 'custom', in the same way that high street shops or supermarkets have to compete with each other and try to do better than the next shop in order to attract customers. Ultimately, if enough patients chose to go elsewhere then a hospital would go bankrupt – although the political consequences of a hospital going 'out of business' are such that we've struggled to know how best to respond to Trusts that are struggling. Later on, high-performing Trusts became designated as **Foundation Trusts**, with greater freedoms and flexibilities to innovate (although these sometimes seemed to exist on paper rather than in reality, with many Foundation Trusts still feeling very heavily controlled by central government/ national bodies).

This system was known as a **quasi-market** or an **internal market**. If I want to buy some shoes, I take my own money and have complete freedom as to which shop I buy from. While the principle is the same with this system, receiving something as complex and fundamental as health care is also arguably very different. Although I may know which shoes I like best, I'm probably not best placed to know what sort of health care I need or what good brain surgery looks like (to take but one example). I'm therefore not a private customer buying goods from a market; instead, I pay my taxes and NHS organisations (**CCGs** in their most recent incarnation) decide what kinds of services are needed for the local population and how best to secure these on my behalf. There is therefore a third party – an NHS commissioner – involved in the process, which isn't the case in a private market (hence the phrase **quasi-market**).

Commissioning is an unusual phrase and tends not be very meaningful in everyday discussion. However, it means deciding what needs exist in a local area, deciding what services might be needed, securing and funding those services, monitoring the quality of what's delivered and seeking feedback to make future improvements. While this system spread throughout the UK, both Wales and Scotland have since retreated from this approach, and they now have a more unified, less competitive system (where the roles of commissioner and provider are combined in a single local organisation). However, in England, the commissioning agenda has raised a series of longstanding questions:

- Is health care the same as other goods or services, and are the mechanisms and concepts associated with a 'market' the best way to design our NHS? This is a highly politicised debate, and different groups tend to have very different but equally strong views.
- Do we have the right skills and can commissioning ever be a strong enough lever to make significant changes in our health services, especially given the size and power of hospitals? While hospital services have tended to remain fairly stable over time, commissioning organisations have been repeatedly reorganised – often in the name of creating a stronger commissioning function, but arguably weakening commissioning in the short term as the new changes bed in.
- Is competition a good way to organise a system, or do we need to find ways of promoting much greater collaboration and integration?
- Following the creation of an **internal market**, the NHS is more of a network or system than it is a single entity or organisation – so who is in charge? With a series of local bodies in competition with each other, and a series of national bodies with different but sometimes overlapping roles, we have now a very fragmented system and it is difficult to see how difficult decisions are meant to be made or how accountability is meant to work.

At the same time as these changes were taking place in the NHS, a similar process was underway in local government and adult social care. Over time, local government had to separate its commissioning and provision functions, putting a number of its in-house services out to tender through regimes known as **compulsory competitive**

tendering and **best value**. Over time, a number of different models have developed, with some councils seeing themselves as 'commissioning-only' and transferring a number of their services out into standalone companies, the voluntary sector or the commercial sector. Other retain some in-house services, but have a strong separation between their commissioning functions and their provider arm. In adult social care, social workers became known as **care managers** and their role shifted from providing a therapeutic service or engaging in community work to assessing people's needs, drawing up a **care plan** with them and deciding which services should meet these needs (in a **care package**). Once again, this required new skills – for example, drawing up and costing out a care plan, then commissioning the different services to provide particular inputs – and there has since been concern that this undermines social work skills and reduces the role to more of a bureaucratic exercise. Even the language employed is interesting – under this system, staff are 'managers' of people's care, rather than 'social workers'. Interestingly, the initial guidance suggested calling social workers 'case managers', but service users resisted this language – in their view they had care needs that could be managed by a worker (if this is how the system wanted to describe it), but they were not 'cases' to be managed.

While the NHS changes took many decades to work through, the transition in local government felt much more rapid. In the early 1990s, local government acquired responsibility for funding nursing and residential care (some of which had previously been paid for in part by the national social security system). For many people, this was an explicit attempt to pass off a rapidly escalating national budget on local councils, knowing that they would have to balance the books and find ways to bring this spending back under control. While councils received funding for their new responsibilities, 85% of this had to be spent in the voluntary or private sectors (a stipulation which – for all the accusations of privatisation – would be unthinkable in the NHS). Over time, this requirement coupled with rising financial pressures meant that the vast majority of social care services are now provided by the private sector (sometimes by large multi-national companies which can be difficult for local councils to scrutinise or influence). While some see this as providing significant economies of scale, others have been highly critical of this fundamental shift (which has arguably taken place without much public debate and without many people realising that this is the case) A strong critic of these changes is Bob Hudson, whose blogs and commentaries have highlighted what he sees as the risks (see **Voices of Experience 3**).

Voices of Experience 3: 'The unsuccessful privatisation of social care'

The shift in the sectoral provision of social care over the last thirty years or so [so that most care is now privatised] is remarkable, and with funding in excess of £22 billion, this is a large and attractive market. In 1979, 64 per cent of residential and nursing home beds were still provided by local authorities or the NHS; by 2012 it was 6 per cent; in the case of domiciliary care, 95 per cent was directly provided by local authorities as late as 1993; by 2012 it was just 11 per cent. This shift to the private sector has also been accompanied by a growing role for large companies with 50+ homes at the expense of small, family-run businesses – five large chains alone now account for 20 per cent of provision and this figure is expected to rise.

Does this matter? The narrative is that users are indifferent to who provides a public service. Instead, it is the quality that matters. But the reality is that the two are inter-twined. The most obvious example is with the workforce which comprises 60 per cent of the costs and is 'sweated' in order to sustain financial margins. Research has highlighted an array of poor practices – restricting annual leave, reducing the numbers of qualified nursing staff, increasing resident-staff ratios, removing sick pay, failing to pay the National Minimum Wage and increased use of zero-hour contracts. Moreover there is evidence that pay rates and staff retention rates are significantly lower in the private sector than in the smaller local authority and voluntary provider sectors.

It would be idle to pretend that this does not impact upon the quality of care. When private care homes are fending off financial problems, the quality of the care that they provide to residents has been found to diminish: the facilities deteriorate, staffing levels are reduced and additional 'services' for residents such as outings or entertainment, are cut back. In the case of domiciliary care there has been wholesale adoption of a flawed 'task and time' model with units of as little as 15 minutes per client imposed in order to reduce costs. And in perhaps the ultimate 'commodification' of care, some local authorities have put care packages for vulnerable people out to tender in eBay-style timed auctions ...

The big private care providers are based upon such fragile and high-risk investments models (designed to maximise short-term financial returns) that they are at risk of market failure. There has already been one spectacular such failure – Southern Cross in 2011 – and a recent survey of local authorities reveals that most are expecting further failure in the coming year. The inappropriate nature of these high-risk financial models premised upon quick and unrealistic returns of 12 per cent on investment has been brilliantly exposed in a report from the Centre for Research in Socio-Cultural Change [www.mbs.ac.uk/news/where-does-the-money-go-when-your-local-authority-pays-more-than-500-per-week-for-a-care-home-bed/]. The bizarre situation now exists whereby some of the biggest private providers of health and care are using tax havens to avoid their fiscal responsibilities and then begging the taxpayer to underwrite their morally dubious investment techniques. The report sensibly proposes a maximum return on investment of 5 per cent ...

Ultimately, however, we need to question the place of large tax-evading private chains founded upon risky financial models having any place in the realm of personal care and support where the free market cannot profitably supply the services needed to meet people's needs. There may well be a place for a mixed economy of small, local private providers and voluntary sector providers alongside a revitalised role for local authorities, but the wholesale dash for privatisation in England cannot be deemed to have been successful in meeting the needs of service users.

Source: Hudson (2016) LSE British Politics and Policy blog

Understanding some of the similarities and differences between health and social care is a key feature of this book – and it is interesting to note that the rapid transformation of adult social care sector was very different to the almost glacial changes that seemed to be taking place in the NHS. There is probably an important cultural issue here – because of its popularity and size and the strength of its professions, the NHS is often really good at paying lip service to the whims of the latest minister but quietly finding ways to carry on as before. In contrast, social work may protest openly and complain significantly, but ultimately ends up doing what it's told. Whether this is a good or a bad thing probably depends on your point of view. If you're a new minister with a brilliant plan to improve services and vested interests within the NHS hold you back and stop patients from benefitting, then these tendencies are incredibly frustrating. Equally, if a minister comes in with a pre-conceived plan that is ill thought through or likely to be damaging then the ability to say "Of course, Minister" then gently ignore her/him is probably a helpful self-protective layer.

A mixed economy of care

A key element of **commissioning** and of public service markets is a **mixed economy of care** from which commissioners can choose services. Once the commissioner has decided what needs exist and what services are required, they can negotiate with different providers to see who might be best to provide what. In England, this can involve having to go out to the market with a 'tender', seeking bids from interested providers and having a transparent process for choosing which provider best meets the commissioner's requirements. In principle, this could be from the public, private or voluntary sectors – what matters is who is best to provide the best service, not where they come from. This notion is well expressed in a book by a former Chief Executive of the NHS (Crisp, 2011, p 91):

> Most NHS staff and members of the public thought of the NHS in terms of the actual bricks and mortar of the hospitals and expected care to be given by NHS employed staff in NHS owned facilities. In the Department [of Health] however we were at this stage starting to think of the NHS as more like a guarantee or a promise of care. The NHS would make sure you were looked after well and got the care you needed whether you were treated in an NHS hospital or a charity or a private one. You would be an NHS patient in every case and entitled to the same standards, rights and privileges and you would access it in the same way through your GP, phone line or Accident and Emergency Department.
>
> Thinking of the NHS in this way … opened up enormous possibilities for innovative services. We were no longer bound by old restrictions as to who might offer a service or how … Funding would continue to come from taxes and services would continue to be available to every citizen according to their need and regardless of their ability to pay. The NHS would continue to be free at the point of need but there would be greater flexibility in the way in which it was delivered.

This provides a fascinating insight into how senior policymakers began to change how they were thinking about public services – moving from a view that public services have to be provided by the public sector, to a view of the public sector as something that arranges care, funds it and guarantees its quality, irrespective of who actually provides it. When members of the public understand this, it usually provokes significant debate. Some people think that public services should be provided by the public sector, and that there are major problems with the quote above (see **Voices of Experience 3** above for an almost diametrically opposed viewpoint). Other people say that they don't care who provides a service as long as it's good.

In many ways, these debates tap into broader political debates about what roles we feel should be played by the public, private and voluntary sectors, and about the assumptions and attitudes we hold about each sector. However, for people new to health and social care, a key thing to remember is that the nature of these debates is probably more complicated than most people realise:

1. Although most people see GPs as a key part of the NHS and as very trusted people, they are often private business people contracting their services to the health service (see Chapter One).
2. Lots of health and social care has always been delivered by very specialist voluntary organisations, who are expert at what they do, highly trusted by the public and leading players in their field. As but one example, hospices are voluntary organisations, part-funded by the NHS and part-funded through donations and fundraising. There are also lots of organisations that specialise in a particular condition (the Alzheimer's Society, the MS Society) as well as voluntary organisations that focus on areas such as mental health and substance misuse.
3. Many hospitals have charities that raise additional funds on their behalf, and many earn additional private income (from both private and international patients) which they reinvest in NHS services. Hospitals in England charge for car parking and can raise significant sums to offset the cost of providing and maintaining these facilities.
4. Lots of services (such as laundry or catering) are contracted out to the commercial sector.
5. Some doctors have contracts working in the public sector, but also undertake additional private work. Similarly, some health and social care staff work for a main employer, but may also be part of an NHS 'bank' that pays them extra to work additional hours, or part of a private agency (which makes its money by recruiting staff to fill NHS vacancies on a temporary basis). Many dentists see a mix of NHS and private patients, and some private

counsellors or physiotherapists may accept NHS referrals but also see paying clients on a private basis.

6. A number of organisations defy easy categorisation – for example, **social enterprises** are voluntary organisations serving charitable aims, but also seek to generate income on a more commercial basis (albeit with a view to reinvesting in their mission). Some services have also moved out of the NHS or local council and set themselves as a staff cooperative providing services for their former employer. Some national or multi-national voluntary organisations may also seem more like large private bodies than they do small, local charities.

7. In adult social care, a number of services are provided by **micro-enterprises** – very small organisations where one or two people (sometimes with experience of using services themselves) support a small number of other part, either on paid or on a voluntary basis.

While concerns about the perceived marketisation of the NHS continue (see, for example, NHS Support Federation, 2017), Powell and Miller (2015, pp 99–100) have argued that the reality may be more nuanced than this:

> Since political devolution in 1998, it has been argued that there are increasing differences between the health services of England, Scotland, Wales and Northern Ireland. For example, Scotland and Wales both disbanded the internal National Health Service … market and have taken a more collaborative (in principle at least) and less competitive approach to their governance and incentives … This has been seen as a fork in the road for privatization … There has been much debate about 'privatizing' the English NHS … The problem is that debate and conclusions require some agreement on basic definitions and on the nature of 'evidence', but this does not appear to be possible at present. This debate (or non-debate) tends to generate more heat than light as definitions and operationalizations of 'privatization' are often implicit, unclear and conflicting, resulting in the term being a general 'boo word' that lacks definitional and analytical precision.

The impact of austerity

Whatever stance different readers take to the themes above, there is no doubt that these issues have got harder and more controversial following the austerity agenda pursued by the Conservative-Liberal Democrat Coalition of 2010–2015 and the Conservative government (2015–). In the late 2000s, the international banking crisis caused shockwaves around the world. As the BBC explains:

On 9 August 2007 we felt the first tremor of a full-blown financial earthquake, whose aftershocks we are still dealing with today – nationally, locally and personally. The crisis ripped a huge hole in the nation's finances as a steep economic downturn caused a sharp fall in government tax receipts. By 2010, the government was having to borrow £1 in every £4 it spent. Although the amount the government is borrowing every year is now falling, the total debt pile is still rising and currently stands at a whopping £1.7 trillion. That's nearly 90% of the UK's total national income.

The financial stress at a national level was soon felt at local level. As the government desperately tried to cut spending, local authorities saw their funding slashed with consequences for the services they provide. Childcare, social care, museums, roads, libraries and others felt the axe fall in the coalition government's controversial austerity drive. Local government spending has fallen 25% in real terms since the crisis.

It's not just public services that felt the impact. Personal incomes have stagnated in the 10 years since the crisis. History tells us that real wages and living standards should rise. In fact, for every £100 taken home 10 years ago, workers are now taking home £97.80 after allowing for inflation. That reality had the Bank of England governor, Mark Carney, reaching for the history books as he recently observed that the UK hasn't seen a period of such weak income growth since the 19th Century. Not all of the income squeeze can be blamed on the crisis. The changing shape of the UK economy – with more jobs created

in lower-paying roles – has played its part, but the wages rot
really set in after the crisis.

The highest level of government debt since the war, swingeing
cuts in public services and falling real incomes. The last ten years
have been unique – and not in a good way. (Jack, 2017)

In the UK, these challenges – arguably beyond the control of any
national government – were faced by the Coalition government
formed in 2010. They believed that a key response to the crisis
should be to cut government spending so that the country could
adapt to these new circumstances and live within its means (just as
a family has to dramatically review and reduce their expenditure if
their financial circumstances suddenly change for the worse). Others
disagreed and argued that the way to recover from such a situation
was to spend more (for example on big infrastructure projects) to
help preserve jobs, taking advantage of low interest rates to help
kickstart the economy. The Conservative Party was also felt to be
ideologically committed to reducing public spending (see Chapter
One for discussion of different political ideologies), and there were
claims by their opponents that they sought to use the financial crisis
as an excuse for making cuts that they would have wanted to make
in any case. The Coalition, for its part, disagreed – retorting that
these were difficult choices that any government would have to make.

For public services, the result has been nearly a decade of cuts and
financial pressures, with seemingly no end in sight (see **Facts and
Figures 8** and **9**). This is very different to the previous decade, when
the UK economy was strong and when the New Labour government
invested heavily in public services (and in health and social care in
particular). During the 2000s, the size of the NHS budget effectively
tripled, with significant investment in staff and facilities. Adult social
care also benefitted significantly, with a series of year-on-year real-
terms increases. From 2010, the Coalition pledged to ringfence the
NHS budget, but ongoing lack of the investment needed meant
financial pressures soon began to spiral out of control. In adult
social care, the cuts to local government funding bit deep, and
there is an ever growing sense of a system in crisis (see **Voices of**

Experience 1 in the Introduction). In practical terms, this means that people who gained their experience and became senior in an era of relative plenty are now having to lead and manage in very different financial circumstances, and it remains to be seen whether we learn to adapt to very challenging financial and service pressures and to what looks like becoming the new normal.

Facts and Figures 8: Adult social care cuts in numbers

£2.5 billion – *the funding gap facing adult social care in 2019–20.*

7% – *the real-terms cut in gross spending on adult social care services by councils, from £19.1 billion in 2009–10 to £17.8 billion in 2016–17.*

25% – *the reduction in the number of older people accessing publicly funded social care, equating to more than 400,000 people, due to tightened eligibility criteria.*

9.5% – *the increase in hours of unpaid care provided between 2009 and 2014.*

1.2 million – *the number of older people estimated to have unmet care needs.*

50 – *the number of councils who have had adult care contracts handed back to them by providers.*

64 – *the number of councils who had experienced the closure of adult care providers in their area.*

6.6% – *the overall staff vacancy rate across adult social care in 2016–17.*

10.4% – *the vacancy rate in domiciliary care in 2016–17.*

95,000 – *the number of people from Europe working in the adult social care sector, compared to 67,000 five years ago.*

£1.3 billion – the amount of money required to stabilise the adult social care provider market.

£366 million – social care overspends reported by councils in 2016–17.

£824 million – savings required in 2017–18.

24% – the proportion of funding authorities in England which say they have enough care provision to meet demand.

Although the government announced an extra £2 billion for adult social care in the Spring Budget, the Local Government Association [LGA] has said this is not enough to deal with all immediate and short-term pressures on adult social care, and highlighted that the funding stops at the end of 2019–20. It also pointed out that this funding was followed by the introduction in July of "further, more rigid and unrealistic target reductions on delayed transfers of care", and the possibility of sanctions if targets were not met.

Although the adult social care council tax precept, which enables local authorities to raise council tax bills by 3% in 2017–18 and a further 3% 2018–19 to help fund adult social care, was a "welcome short-term measure", the LGA said extra council tax income "will not bring in anywhere near enough money to alleviate the growing pressure on social care both now and in the future".

It also said the government's main vehicle for driving integration, the Better Care Fund (BCF), had "lost credibility and is no longer fit for purpose". Its focus on reducing pressure on NHS acute services "is detracting from local initiatives to support social care and stabilise the perilously fragile social care provider market."

Source: Social care's funding pressures in numbers, Community Care, 21 November 2017, www.communitycare.co.uk/2017/11/21/social-cares-funding-crises-numbers/). Full references can be found in the source material at www.communitycare.co.uk.

Facts and Figures 9: Financial pressures on the NHS

In autumn 2017, three leading thinktanks/charities, the Nuffield Trust, the Health Foundation and the King's Fund (2017, pp 3–6), published a briefing on the financial pressures facing health and social care. The quotes below are long and detailed – but the key messages are really important:

- *Seven years of austerity and rising demand for services is taking a mounting toll on patient care. Waiting times are rising, with patient rights under the NHS Constitution routinely breached; access to some services is being restricted; general practice, mental health and community services are under huge pressure.*
- *The amount the government currently plans to spend is not enough to maintain standards of care and meet the rising demand for health services. 2018/19 will be a crunch year for the NHS with funding growth slowing to just 0.4 per cent, the lowest rate of growth of this parliament and one of the lowest in NHS history.*
- *... We estimate that NHS spending would need to rise from £123.8 billion to at least £153 billion between 2017/18 and 2022/23 (a 4.3 per cent average annual increase) to keep pace with demographic pressures and other increasing cost pressures.*
- *On current spending plans, we estimate that NHS spending would increase to only £128.4 billion in 2022/23 (a 0.7 per cent average annual increase). This falls a long way short of what is needed.*
- *Throughout this parliament there will be a significant and growing gap between the resources given to the NHS and the demands it faces. In 2018/19 alone, we estimate that NHS spending will be at least £4 billion lower than the level required.*

The NHS does not have the resources it needs to maintain access to high-quality patient care

An unprecedented seven-year funding squeeze and rising demand for services are taking a mounting toll on patient care. The Care Quality Commission (CQC) 2017 State of Care report warns that health and care services are at full stretch and that some services have deteriorated. There is also growing evidence that access to some treatments is being rationed and that quality of care in some services is being diluted. All areas of care are affected, with acute hospitals, general practice, mental health and community services under strain.

Key waiting time standards are now being missed all year round, and the deterioration in performance shows few signs of stopping. The four-hour standard for treating patients in A&E has not been met since July 2015; the 62-day standard for beginning treatment for cancer following an urgent referral has not been met for more than three years; the 18-week referral-to-treatment target for planned care has not been met since February 2016 and has been given lower priority from March 2017. In July 2017, nearly 900 patients with acute mental health needs were inappropriately placed outside their local area due to a lack of available local inpatient beds. Patient satisfaction with GP services has dropped from 88.4 per cent in June 2012 to 84.8 per cent in July 2017, while in a recent survey, more than half of GP practices said that pressures are so great they would consider temporarily preventing new patients from registering with them.

The CQC notes that the quality of care that patients actually receive across England is mostly good. This is due to the efforts of NHS staff in delivering compassionate care in challenging circumstances. But this resilience is limited and the situation increasingly precarious. Without additional funding, the NHS will not be able to achieve the commitments made to patients in the NHS Constitution.

The implications of the funding squeeze on patients' access to care are already clear – the dramatic improvements achieved over the previous two decades, which were hard fought and required considerable investment, are now slipping away. If this is not rectified, patients will wait longer to access the urgent and routine clinical care they need.

Whatever happens next to health and social care funding, there are a number of key themes and hot topics that are helping to shape the future of UK services:

1. *Financial and service pressures:* both health and social care are facing the twin challenges of rising need/demand and financial pressures (a mixture of active cuts, budgets remaining flat and/or budgets failing to keep pace with demand). In adult social care, this means that more people are in need but that fewer people are getting support, and that those who do qualify for publicly funded services receive less support than in the past. In the NHS, there are record numbers of people seeking help and the service has been systematically failing to meet both waiting time targets and financial targets for some time. Across the board, some services are closing altogether, some treatments are being cut back and service pressures are increasing.

2. *Workforce and other challenges:* these pressures are not merely financial: often, services respond to funding shortages by cutting anything that will not immediately harm frontline services (including education and training budgets). This is entirely understandable but usually proves to be false economy in the longer term, with significant workforce shortages building up across the whole of the NHS and social care. As but one example, the NAO (2018) has published a highly critical report on the adult social care workforce, highlighting high turnover and vacancy rates, rising demand for care, significant recruitment and retention problems (with care work seen as low pay and low skilled) and the complete absence of an up-to-date workforce strategy. When money is tight, we also usually cut back on our

spending equipment and estates – and this can create long-term backlogs which are difficult to overcome. While spending on equipment can feel frivolous in very challenged financial times, lots of equipment in the NHS in particular is quite literally life-saving – and scrimping on this isn't the right thing to do. Similarly, if we don't invest in our estate for a prolonged period of time, then we may need to spend even more to bring buildings back up to standard than if we'd funded smaller amounts of upkeep and maintenance on a regular basis.

3. *Sustainability of care markets:* in adult social care, there are widespread concerns about the level of fees that local councils can pay to service providers, with some services worrying that they cannot afford to keep going or that they are having to compromise significantly on quality. There are also a series of unanswered questions about how we fund increased costs (such as the National Living Wage, equal pay claims and the wages of people who are sleeping over within residential services – who might previously have been paid a flat rate for this, but should have been paid at least the minimum wage).

4. *Misaligned financial incentives:* in the NHS in England, the logic of **Payment by Results** is that hospitals should be adequately paid for everyone they treat (so that if they provide a really good service and more people choose to go to that hospital rather than another, the money follows the choice of the patient). In practice, there have been concerns that this could encourage hospitals to admit people rather than support **care closer to home**, and so the fee per patient is reduced beyond a certain level of activity (often based on historic patient numbers rather than current demand). However, with rapidly increasing levels of need, this means that good hospitals who are attracting patients don't feel that they are adequately funded for the patients they are seeing – and that they get financially penalised for being popular/providing good care. Others would argue that hospitals get over-funded compared to other parts of the health and social care system, so that they may just need to get over it. Wherever the truth lies, the risk is that we spend longer on internal debates about what commissioners

should or shouldn't be paying providers, and less on trying to keep people healthy and out of hospital in the first place.

5. *Efficiencies:* in both health and social care, services are responding to the financial challenges they face by seeking major efficiencies in terms of how they deliver current services: in local government, these decisions are (by definition) locally based, and individual councils are negotiating with local people and their own directorates as to what budget they set and which services have to save how much money in order to balance the books. In the NHS, there have been a series of attempts to articulate the total efficiencies that may be needed if the service is to continue to meet rising needs. For example, under the leadership of Sir David Nicholson, the NHS pursued a policy of Quality, Innovation, Productivity and Prevention (QIPP), seeking to achieve savings of around £20 billion between 2010 and 2015 in order to respond to the challenges facing the health service. This quickly became known as 'the Nicholson challenge' and, unfortunately, often seemed to be reduced to attempts to generate savings, rather than a more fundamental exploration of how increased quality, greater prevention and more innovative approaches could enhance productivity. More recently, the *NHS Five Year Forward View* identified the need for an additional £30 billion by 2020/21, with one of the options set out assuming £8 billion extra funding per year and £22 billion of efficiency savings (NHS England, 2014) – a challenging set of assumptions, to say the least! Unfortunately, this seems to have led to a situation where the government is claiming it is giving the NHS what it asked for, and the NHS is claiming the government hasn't – with significant tension and mutual recriminations.

The funding of long-term care

In the midst of all these funding challenges is a longstanding debate about how to fund long-term care (24-hour residential and nursing home care) for older people. Although this is currently under review in England, this is thought to be the 13th consultation or official policy paper on this topic over the past 20 years – and none have yet been fully implemented. One of the difficulties is that many people assume that care homes are funded in the same way as the NHS, and that care is free at the point of delivery. In fact, care homes are funded by local authorities (for people who meet eligibility criteria and qualify on financial grounds), and many people have to pay towards the cost of their care. This calculation is based not just on savings and income, but also on the cost of people's homes (see **Key Sources 1**) – and so anyone who owns their own property can find themselves having to sell their home (or place a charge on it to be recovered after their death), paying substantial weekly sums. In practice, local authorities funding someone's care have usually negotiated a much lower rate for publicly funded care, with homes cross-subsidising this by charging much higher rates to people funding their own care. For someone wanting to go into a care home that is more expensive than the local council is prepared to pay, a third party (usually a family member) has to agree to pay the difference. Where someone lives with a partner, a child under 18 or a relative who is over 60 or disabled, the cost of someone's home isn't taken into account.

Key Sources 1: Paying for a care home

How much will I have to pay for care?

Care home fees will vary depending on the area that you live in, the individual care home itself, plus your own personal financial circumstances.

Your local authority must calculate the cost of your care and how much you have to contribute from your resources. This figure must be realistic and allow you to access an appropriate local care home.

If all your eligible income is taken into account in your means-test, you must be left with an income of £24.90 per week. This is known as your Personal Expenses Allowance ...

How could my finances and property affect my care home fees?

If your local authority carries out a care needs assessment and finds you need a care home place, they will do a means test. This may take into account the value of your property, if you own one, as well as your income and savings. Here's how the means test for social care will look at your capital and how this will affect your care home fees.

Amount of your capital (your savings and property)	What you will have to pay
Over £23,250	You must pay full fees (known as being self-funding)
Between £14,250 and £23,250	The local authority will pay for some of your care and you will contribute to the rest
Less than £14,250	This will be ignored and won't be included in the means-test – the local authority will pay for your care. However they will still take your eligible income into account

Source: Paying for a care home, Age UK, www.ageuk.org.uk/information-advice/care/care-homes/paying-for-a-care-home/

According to *Which?*, the independent consumer champion:

In 2016–17, the average weekly cost of a room in a residential home in the UK was £600, and a room in a nursing home cost £841. However, these are only average figures, so you or your relative could be looking at considerably higher or lower figures depending on where you live. (www.which.co.uk/ elderly-care/financing-care/financing-a-care-home/381597-care-home-fees)

For older people and their families suddenly discovering this reality (often in a crisis and when feeling really unwell or vulnerable), it can come as a complete shock and feels like a betrayal of the promises that people think were made for the welfare state to care for them from the cradle to the grave. This has generated significant anger and protest, often focusing on the extent to which people should be able to pass on their homes to their families after they die, or whether they should be expected to sell these homes to pay for their care. This is particularly difficult in situations where older people are 'cash poor but asset rich'. For example, where I grew up in Devon, there were frail older people with no real money, but living in houses worth many hundreds and hundreds of thousands of pounds, which would be completely out of reach for a younger generation struggling to afford to live in the local area. This raises all sorts of complex issues about who should pay for what, about what we should prepare for while we are working in terms of future care costs, about different pressures in different areas of the country, and about fairness and equity between generations. There are also debates as to whether we should have the same solution for everyone with significant care needs, or whether people with a life-long impairment and who need a care home throughout their adult lives should be funded differently to older people who become frail in later life. While some people say that the latter should have been able to prepare for future care costs, others feel that such older people have already paid a lifetime of taxes and shouldn't have to pay a second time. Many people also argue that no one knows in advance who is going to incur significant care costs in later life (for example, if someone develops dementia and spends a number of years in a care home) compared to those of us who may die suddenly and not need caring for at all. This can quickly become a very polarised debate, with those who are against property taxes claiming that taking people's homes into account (perhaps selling these after someone has died) is a form of 'death tax', while others claim that the current system is effectively a 'dementia tax'.

Every time the issue is reviewed, a very logical, coherent solution is put forward – only for this to prove too politically unpalatable/ unpopular and for the latest proposals to be shelved. This has happened on multiple occasions, and recent debates feel to many like a case of history repeating itself. Interestingly, the situation in Scotland is very different to England, with the Scottish Executive choosing to implement the proposals produced by the 1999 Royal Commission on Long Term Care (the first major review under the New Labour government – see Dickinson and Glasby, 2006, for further discussion). This suggested providing **free personal care** to people in residential and nursing homes (so that care is free to people in the same way it would be if they were in hospital) – but with people contributing towards their housing and living costs (the equivalent of the food and rent/mortgage that people would be paying for if they weren't in a care home). Although the funding of long-term care is often seen as an economic issue (how much can we afford to pay?), the experience in Scotland shows that these are ultimately political choices. While England decided that the proposals from the Royal Commission were unaffordable, Scotland felt they were a price worth paying for what they saw as a fairer, better system. Ultimately, we are unlikely to resolve these longstanding national debates without greater public debate and consensus about what quality of care we want to provide for older people, how much we're collectively prepared to pay for this, and the best mechanisms for bringing this about.

The personalisation agenda

Earlier in this chapter we saw how health and social care (in England at least) have placed greater emphasis on **commissioning** as a way of improving care. Much of this discussion was about strategic commissioning (deciding what services an entire area or local population might need). However, this agenda was in many ways pre-dated by a focus on what might be described as a form of 'micro-commissioning' – with individual disabled people given access to care funding with which to design and control their own support. The origins of these ideas (currently described as a form of 'self-directed support' or as a **personalisation agenda**) have been set out in much greater detail elsewhere (Glasby and Littlechild, 2016), but two of the key concepts are:

- **Direct payments**: where individual disabled people receive direct funds with which to purchase their own care from a private or voluntary agency, or to hire their own care staff (often called 'personal assistants').

- **Personal budgets**: where the worker is clear upfront how much is available to spend on meeting the person's assessed need and where the person has a choice about how this money is spent on their behalf. While this could be via a direct payment, it could also be via the local authority retaining the money on the person's behalf but spending it in a mutually agreed way, or with the money being controlled by a friend, a family member, a service provider or a broker.

Although beginning in adult social care, both concepts have since spread to the NHS, so that people with particular health needs (or with both health and social care needs) can benefit from these ways of working (see Further resources, at the end of this chapter).

The crucial thing about this agenda is that **direct payments** in particular were invented by disabled people, who wanted to have greater control over their services and hence over their lives. They were initially brought across to the UK from the US and Canada in the early 1980s by small groups of disabled people lobbying their local councils. These were often young people in wheelchairs who were living in residential care, but wanted to be able to design more innovative care arrangements that would enable them to live independently in the community. As these ideas spread, there was a concerted campaign to get this way of working taken up and promoted by government, and direct payments finally became part of national policy via the Community Care (Direct Payments) Act 1996. More recently, successive governments have championed the separate – but linked – notion of **personal budgets**, and all adult social care is now meant to be delivered in this way (except in an emergency).

This is an exciting but controversial agenda, and many areas have struggled to implement these ideas in a way which is consistent with their underlying value base. For some people, this could represent a further privatisation of social care (and now of the NHS too), damaging public sector services and ethos. For others, this is a debate about citizenship and human rights, with disabled people having the same right to choice and control as non-disabled people.

Where these mechanisms have tended to work really well, there have usually been disabled people who are angry at the lack of choice and control they have, staff keen to find a way to use scarce public resources in a more imaginative way, local organisations of disabled people campaigning for change and providing peer support, and local leaders ready to champion new ideas. Where things have worked badly, it's been because we have an under-funded system, with demoralised staff and a lack of leadership, only paying lip service to notions of choice and control and using the new language as a smokescreen for cuts. Direct payments and personal budgets have therefore been described a 'Marmite' issue: deep down, people either love them or hate them (see Needham and Glasby, 2014, for further discussion; see also **Voices of Experience 4** for practical examples of **personalisation** in action).

Voices of Experience 4: Personal health budgets

"At the age of five I was diagnosed with Duchenne Muscular Dystrophy, a condition causing my muscles to get progressively weaker. When I was 12 my Dad left work to become my full time carer because I rapidly began to need more and more support with day to day life. This worked well for numerous years. The difficulties began as I entered adulthood. As an adult I needed to have choice and control over my daily life, but I was totally reliant on my Dad to get out, socialise and do activities I enjoyed. He had his own life to lead and responsibilities to take care of and so wasn't always able to enable me to do what I wanted. Having no independence led me to feel depressed and isolated. I now have a Personal Health Budget which I use to employ PAs [personal assistants] to care for me 24/7 and it's had a huge impact on me. I have grown in confidence by taking on new responsibilities and having greater choice and control has given me new self-esteem and an increased appetite for life." (Tom)

"I had a spinal injury in 2006 ... which left me needing 24 hour care. When I came home from hospital, I had a joint-funded

traditional live-in care package delivered by a specialist spinal injury care agency. I moved to a PHB [personal health budget] in 2015 with a direct payment, which enabled me, for the first time, to take control of my care – and my life! Being able to choose the people who support me, to live my life the way that I want to, has completely transformed my whole life. I'm no longer worrying about whether the next PA will be able to get me out of bed safely, let alone out of the house and instead am back working, with an active social life, and am enjoying being able to be myself again." (Robyn)

"My dad, Malcolm, started receiving his personal health budget in 2009. Three years previous he had begun displaying symptoms of early onset dementia and by 2009, his needs were very complex. He had a rare form of dementia – right frontal lobe, which meant it was difficult to anticipate what changes in behaviour and needs he might display and because of this, suitable support packages were difficult to find. Having a personal health budget provided consistency in his care. He employed 5 PAs who supported him in his own home. He was also able to continue enjoying hobbies that kept him stimulated such as going to football, to the cinema and for walks. The package was also a win/win for the NHS, saving an estimated £100k a year compared to care home costs in an assessment made in 2014. Because of his personal health budget, he was able to stay living at home for the rest of his life." (Colin)

"I have Motor Neurone Disease. It's a usually terminal, rapidly progressing, degenerative disease that well over 60% of people diagnosed with, die within 14 months. It's a horrendous death, all the muscles wasting away and eventually the breathing muscle (diaphragm) stops working and we die. Around 85% of people die within three years and only a very small percentage live beyond 5 years. I have consistently beaten the prognoses because the care I get is personalised and has one goal, keeping me alive, healthy, independent and nourished, both physically and mentally. It's safe to say that without a personal health budget and Continuing Health

Care, I would have died several years ago. What best describes my experience of having a personal health budget? Simple really, Life, and having the support to squeeze every last drop of living, out of however much time I have left." (Keith)

Source: All stories provided by peoplehub (see www.peoplehub.org.uk for more examples and information) – see also www.england.nhs.uk/personal-health-budgets/phbs-in-action/patient-stories/ for further examples

Looking back at this chapter as a whole, it might seem surprising that such in-depth discussion of funding should be so prominent in a book about care. However, the way in which services are funded, how money moves around the system and who controls it are all key issues when it comes to trying to use the funding available to the best possible effect. While money isn't why most people choose to work in health and social care, it still matters – and understanding these topics is important for all of us (as taxpayers, voters and citizens, as well as people who might use and/or work in health and social care).

Further resources

The King's Fund provides an excellent website on **how the NHS is funded** (www.kingsfund.org.uk/publications/how-health-care-is-funded), which includes information on topics such as taxation, private insurance and user charges, as well as on approaches to funding health systems in other countries. They also provide a **'Bite Size' guide to adult social care**, including a short video on how it is funded (www.kingsfund.org.uk/projects/what-is-social-care).

A number of leading thinktanks have produced recent research and policy papers on **health and/or adult social care finances**, including:

- The Health Foundation (www.health.org.uk/collection/research-and-analysis-nhs-funding-and-finances)
- The Institute of Fiscal Studies (www.ifs.org.uk/publications/9186)
- The Nuffield Trust (www.nuffieldtrust.org.uk/spotlight/nhs-finances)

The **Association of Directors of Adult Social Services** publishes a helpful annual budget survey (www.adass.org.uk/ adass-budget-survey-2017).

A key thinker and writer about **quasi–markets** and the **role of choice and competition** is Julian Le Grand (2003, 2007; Le Grand and Bartlett, 1993), who is a leading academic and a former health advisor to Tony Blair during his time as prime minister.

In terms of **commissioning**, *Commissioning for Health and Well-being* (Glasby, 2012) is an edited introductory textbook.

Martin Powell and Robin Miller have written perceptively (and humorously) about ongoing debates around the extent to which the NHS is being privatised and free health care as we know it is about to end (they describe this as 'seventy years of privatizing the British National Health Service' and, tongue in cheek, ask 'who killed the English National Health Service?'; Powell, 2015; Powell and Miller, 2014, 2015). Martin Powell (2007) is also the editor of *Understanding the Mixed Economy of Welfare*.

For the politics and impact of **austerity**, see:

- Bochel, H. and Powell, M. (eds) (2016) *The Coalition Government and Social Policy*, Bristol: Policy Press.
- Exworthy, M., Mannion, R. and Powell, M. (eds) (2016) *Dismantling the NHS? Evaluating the Impact of Health Reforms*, Bristol: Policy Press.
- The Social Policy Association's *In Defence of Welfare* (Foster et al, 2015, www.social-policy.org.uk/wordpress/wp-content/ uploads/2015/04/IDOW-Complete-text-4-online_secured-compressed.pdf).

Charities such as Age UK have excellent factsheets and websites explaining how the **funding of long-term care** works in practice (see, for example, www.ageuk.org.uk/information-advice/care/care-homes/paying-for-a-care-home). There have been various reviews of the funding of long-term care over the past 20 years, including:

- The Royal Commission on Long Term Care (Sutherland, 1999)
- The Wanless Review (2006) – including consideration of the introduction of free personal care in Scotland (Dickinson and Glasby, 2006; Dickinson et al, 2007)
- The Dilnot Review (2011)
- The Barker Review (2014)

A paper on funding options is available from the Health Foundation/ King's Fund (Wenzel, 2018). Internationally, the OECD has published a review of the challenges facing the funding of long-term care (Colombo et al, 2011).

For resources on **direct payments**, **personal budgets** and **personalisation**, see:

- The websites of partnerships/organisations such as Think Local Act Personal (TLAP) (www.thinklocalactpersonal.org.uk), In Control (www.in-control.org.uk) and the Centre for Welfare Reform (www.centreforwelfarereform.org);
- NHS England's framework for personalised health and care (www. england.nhs.uk/personalised-health-and-care-framework);
- Introductory textbooks by Glasby and Littlechild (2016), Needham and Glasby (2014) and Alakeson (2014).

For personal health budgets, there are really powerful and practical stories available via peoplehub's Personal Health Budgets Network (www.peoplehub.org.uk/category/stories).

3

Organising health and social care

In Chapter One we saw how the evolution of policy over time created a series of '*inheritances*' (Greener, 2008, p 10) which have shaped subsequent service delivery and what is possible to achieve or do differently at any given moment of time. This has included a series of potential tensions in terms of the organisation of care between:

- the local, regional and national;
- hospitals, community services and primary care;
- physical and mental health;
- health and social care;
- medical cure and public health/prevention.

Each of these themes is explored in more detail below, before concluding with a short section on current service reconfigurations and service pressures.

The danger of structural solutions

Before moving on to each of the tensions set out above, a key issue to address upfront is the tendency of the NHS in particular to try to deal with some of these issues via repeated structural reorganisations. Given the political importance of the NHS, these can look like a new minister or government is doing something big and bold, sweeping away previous problems and ushering in a new, improved system. However, the reality is such changes probably make things worse in the short term and seem to do little to improve overall outcomes or performance (and then are quickly replaced with a new reorganisation and a new system). Indeed, the title of a blog by Greener (2018) to help celebrate the 50th anniversary of the Social Policy Association argues that 'more funding, not reorganisations, make the NHS better for us all'. Echoing themes from throughout this book, Greener is clear that:

> By 2018 we've had 50 years of NHS reorganisation. Mostly, it hasn't really made things better. Indeed, it is hard to see what much of it was actually for. We still haven't managed to find a way of overcoming the tensions of the tripartite split [between hospital services, primary care and community health services]. We know we need more collaboration between local government and the NHS, especially as the demands on social care services increase and the lack of funding for it has real consequences for services currently paid for by the NHS. However, for many of us, the boundary between health and social care is an artificial one that does not serve our needs.
>
> What does seem to have made a difference is increased funding for the NHS, in real terms, in the 2000s, when a range of measured improvements came along soon after. These improvements are now in danger of disappearing in the austere environment of the 2010s. If there is a big lesson from the history of the last 50 years, it is that health reorganisations often do as much bad as good, but increasing funding for the NHS has a much better chance of improving healthcare for us all.

Similarly, Edwards reviews lessons from previous NHS and other reorganisations, describing the belief that the next reorganisation will work when previous ones didn't as a 'triumph of hope over experience'. Walshe (2003, p 108) reaches a similar conclusion, arguing that:

> There is little point in investing in the long-term development of NHS organizations because they do not usually have a

long term—and so the NHS more and more resembles an organizational shantytown in which structures and systems are cobbled together or thrown up hastily in the knowledge that they will be torn down again in due course.

According to this analysis, the NHS has been engaged in 'a state of almost continuous reform and restructuring' (p 106) for decades, with significant negative implications:

1. Most reforms don't work out as intended, and yet we're often on to the next set of changes before we have fully learned the lessons from the previous reorganisation.
2. Reorganisations take a huge amount of time and effort, and divert attention away from improving frontline services.
3. Reforms are often circular, so similar ideas and structures recur over time and we often end up back where we started.
4. We often forget 'the unhealthy cumulative effects of all this reform on the NHS and its culture'. Indeed, constant change 'engenders a deeply cynical and dismissive attitude to any innovation and change – "we've seen it all before, nothing works, just ignore it and keep your head down because it won't last very long" – which makes the advancement of real changes in health services much more difficult'. (p 108)

As Walshe concludes:

Paradoxically, the more things change, the more they stay the same. None of this bewildering succession of health service reforms has changed the fundamental governance and accountability arrangements of the NHS. The service remains, just as it was when it was founded in 1948, a vertically integrated public bureaucracy run from Whitehall. Despite repeated changes in the labels on the boxes on the organizational chart— regional, district, area and strategic health authorities, family practitioner committees, family health services authorities, NHS Trusts, primary care groups, primary care trusts, and so on—the lines of accountability still run in one direction only, upwards, to the Department of Health and the Secretary of State for Health. The ceaseless reorganization of the NHS can perhaps best be understood as a fruitless search for a way to manage the unmanageable. No organization with a turnover of over £70 billion a year can be run from its central office by administrative diktat, yet that is how generations of politicians have tried to run the NHS. (Walshe, 2003, p 108)

These are strong critiques – and we may well be better off trying to improve current services as best we can, finding ways to manage across boundaries and deal with tensions, rather than resorting to frequent reorganisations. Unfortunately, this is a lesson that NHS policymakers have failed to learn, and there seems little sign that the ongoing organisational churn in the health service will reduce.

Local v regional v national

The 'N' in 'NHS' stands for national, and overall funding is agreed and policy set out at a national level. However, we have already seen in Chapter One how health care is devolved to the four countries of the UK and how structures and approaches differ. With developments in England often dominating the media and debates in Westminster, a lot of what we call the 'national' is often really about England. Each year, the government sets a **mandate** for NHS England (setting out government objectives and any specific requirements for the NHS, as well as the NHS budget). NHS England is then responsible for using this money to deliver these objectives and to arrange the provision of health services (whether through funding and arranging specialist services itself, or distributing funds to local **CCGs** to commission local services). A national inspectorate – the Care Quality Commission – is the independent regulator of health and social care services in England, while NHS Improvement is responsible for overseeing NHS **Foundation Trusts**. At local level, **CCGs** commission local health services from a **mixed economy of care** (see Chapter Two), and GPs and **NHS Trusts** deliver a range of primary, community, mental health and hospital services. While many people assume the Secretary of State is directly responsible for the delivery of health services and that the NHS is a single organisation, responsibility and accountability are actually very complex and fragmented, and the NHS is more of a 'system' than an organisation. As we have already seen in Chapter One, adult social care is organised by local councils, and so approaches differ from area to area (there are 152 councils with social services responsibility in England).

For present purposes, there are four key issues for us to consider here:

1. *The role of politics:* at various stages, a number of different commentators have suggested that there is too much direct political intervention (some would describe it as 'interference' or even as 'tinkering') in the health service. This has led to various attempts to give the NHS more independence from government, balancing the legitimate democratic right of national political leaders to set NHS priorities with the need for NHS organisations and local leaders to have the autonomy they need to deliver against these priorities. Indeed, the creation of NHS England during the Lansley reforms of 2010–12 was the latest in an attempt to create greater independence and a more arms-length relationship between government and the NHS. In practice, the NHS is so important to the public and politically, and receives so much public funding, that politicians will probably always want to have a significant say over what happens in the health service. Moreover, politicians tend to get directly blamed by the public and the media for things that we want changing about the NHS, so there is a natural tendency to want to be able to influence what happens if you're going to be held to account for it (irrespective of whether it's actually your fault or not).

2. *Local responsiveness v economies of scale:* built into this system, and to a series of organisational reforms over time, has been a dilemma between delivering economies of scale (through larger, more regional approaches) and being locally responsive (really

knowing local communities and tailoring services according). Over time, NHS reforms have tended to move backwards and forwards between these two ends of the spectrum, with some reforms creating strong regional bodies and larger organisations, only to be swept away and replaced with more local bodies. After a period of time, a future government will usually decide that there are too many local bodies and that we could make better use of scarce resource and get a better overview of the range of the services needed by different communities if we merged current organisations and created larger bodies. In practice, this is rarely a sensible conversation, and it might be better if we decided what was best to do at individual level, what at local level, what at regional level and what at national level – with different activities best located at different geographical scales (rather than assuming there is a 'perfect organisational structure' waiting for us to find).

3. *The role of the region*: at various stages there has been a regional tier of organisation, seeking to receive national policies and support local delivery, while also providing a regional overview. An example of these (in England) were the Strategic Health Authorities (SHAs) abolished in 2012. While many local health services used to complain that there was too much regional oversight of what they did by the SHA, the abolition of this regional tier has created much more fragmentation and made it harder to coordinate activity across different local partners. A more recent attempt to create greater regional leadership comes via **Sustainability and Transformation Partnerships** (STPs), but the current health care system in England remains very fragmented.

4. *Complexity of interagency boundaries*: health is organised on a national basis (to an extent), while social care is organised locally – and this is a key barrier to more effective joint working. Moreover, at local level, health and social care practitioners can find themselves having to work with a bewildering array of different partner organisations depending on local geography and structures and on exactly where the individual service user lives. When I was training as a social worker, our office might work with five or

six different hospitals, two different mental health providers, two different community health providers, four different groups of GPs and hundreds of individual GP practices, each of which had different policies, budgets, structures and priorities. Equally, a large hospital in our city could find itself liaising with adult social care organised by seven or eight different councils, each with different eligibility criteria, services and contact numbers. Faced with such complexity, getting anything done across agency boundaries could be a major logistical undertaking – and this structure certainly wasn't conducive to quick outcomes or effective two-way relationships with key partners.

Hospitals v community services v primary care

As set out in Chapter One, the NHS has historically been based on a **tripartite system**, with different approaches to the organisation of hospitals, community health and primary care services. In particular, a key concern has been that hospitals have too often been the main focus, consuming the most resources, dominating provision and encouraging a mindset that hospital should be the default option when we're ill. It's certainly easy to see why this might be the case. Anyone who has worked in a hospital can't help but be amazed by the complexity, the hustle and bustle, the expertise and the miraculous things that we're able to do to cure and heal people, 24 hours a day, 7 days a week, 365 days a year. Hospitals are rightly popular with local people, and the visual symbol of our NHS.

However, hospitals often aren't very nice places to be if you don't really need the services provided there. They can be hot, noisy, impersonal and stressful – and people can be at risk of hospital-acquired infections, losing their independence and becoming stuck in a system that has to balance care for the individual with the need to process thousands of people every day. Once someone is over the worst of their illness or injury then they usually want to be able to go home and to get back to some sort of normality in a place where they feel comfortable and at ease. Moreover, lots of conditions that previously needed someone to go to hospital can now be treated safely and appropriately in the community, either in a GP surgery or even in someone's own home. There is also a lot of equipment to help monitor people's health (known as 'telehealth') so that they can stay at home rather than needing to be in a hospital bed for observation. Finally, there has been a longstanding desire to make best use of expensive, scarce resources by only admitting people to hospital beds when absolutely necessary, and to find ways to care for more people in the community.

More recently, this has been described as a desire to promote **care closer to home** – and it's been a remarkably enduring policy aim (although also very hard to achieve in practice) (see **Voices of Experience 5**). To genuinely shift care from one setting to another, you probably need significant investment in new services while you continue to run the previous service, and you need to work long and hard to bring about significant cultural change. Moreover, care closer to home can also be controversial, and can easily be misunderstood by the media or local people. For example, if I develop a new service in the community or in someone's home, this could be viewed by some as being less safe than being in hospital. I might also need to take some money from the hospital budget to invest in community alternatives, hoping that this would one day lead to a reduction in people needing to go to hospital (but probably needing the hospital to treat the same number of people in the mean time). At the same time, the desire to create care closer to home has also been accompanied in some specialties by a desire to create much larger, regional, specialist services – which can be staffed by very senior, experienced people and provide care 24 hours a day (children's heart surgery has been a recent and controversial example). While reformers might feel that this will lead to safer services, local people in an area whose service is being centralised would experience this as a loss – and might suspect that this was the result of cuts rather than a desire to improve care. Thus, how much care we deliver at home and how we organise specialist services can have a significant impact on how we organise local hospital services. Once again, these tensions go right back to the beginning of the NHS, and there is a very powerful quote from Aneurin Bevan that perfectly illustrates some of these tensions:

Many of the hospitals are too small – very much too small. About 70 per cent have less than 100 beds, and over 30 per cent have less than 30. No one can possibly pretend that hospitals so small can provide general hospital treatment. There is a tendency in some quarters to defend the very small hospital on the ground of its localism and intimacy, and for other rather imponderable reasons of that sort, but everybody knows today that if a hospital is to be efficient it must provide a number of specialised services. Although I am not myself a devotee of bigness for bigness sake, I would rather be kept alive in the efficient if cold altruism of a large hospital than expire in a gush of warm sympathy in a small one. (Bevan, 1946)

Voices of Experience 5: Care closer to home: the example of district nursing

As a staff nurse in hospital many years ago, during a particularly trying shift, I heard myself say to a relative who was late "well it isn't actually visiting time – but alright then" and immediately thought, "who do you think you are to stop people visiting their loved ones? – what's the matter with you?" This thought translated into a desire to move out of hospital care, where the needs of the patient could seem secondary to the smooth running of the organisation at times, despite all the kind and well-meaning staff working within the system.

Outside of hospitals, professionals work with people and their daily lives, in their own homes/settings, with their rules. No banning of visitors – even four-legged ones. Indeed you might have to suspend your infection control procedures and try to work around the dog sniffing at the sterile dressings pack if that was the only way the patient would let you near – risk management at a whole new level!

Hospitals play a key role in the NHS and have moved considerably to develop more patient-centred approaches – with open visiting times one such example. At the same time the needs of patients in the community continues to evolve, and more and more complex patients are managed at home: frail elderly patients with multiple long-term conditions; intravenous therapies; people with dementia; and even ventilated patients. And yet the narrative which positions hospital care as the most important aspect of the NHS persists. Compare the wholescale movement of district nursing services from [former Primary Care Trusts] and Community Trusts into a variety of organisations, with the changes or movement of services out of hospitals. Some were moved into private companies or social enterprises. I saw no headlines, petitions or public protests for the former but ubiquitous news coverage of the latter. Hospital pressures regularly feature as newsworthy items – the rise in activity and "winter pressures" seem familiar terms to many of the general population (if my mum is the benchmark!). However, how many people could talk about the pressures which community services are facing?...

It is highly likely that the STPs currently being produced in England, will have a continued focus on providing care outside of hospital, and integrating care around the needs of patients, and not the organisations. This space is one in which the community nursing workforce already operates, and they would have much experience and expertise to share but any additional workload coming their way as a result of the Plans needs to be accommodated somehow.

Whilst Health Education England have developed an education strategy and are beginning to redress the decrease in training places for district nurses there is still much more work to do. There is a real sense of urgency that we need to find, nurture, develop and protect our district nurses – without this, the routine delivery of more services and care closer to home remains a fairy tale … Personally, I like my stories to have a happy ending but I'm still waiting for the hero of the story to be revealed.

Source: Sawbridge (2016) Birmingham University Health Services Management Centre blog.

Physical v mental health

Different cultures define mental ill health in different ways — but western societies have tended to separate physical and mental health (one to do with the body and one to do with the mind). To this day, we still have different specialities and services working with physical and mental health, and the tendency has been for mental health services to lose out in terms of funding, status and public understanding (see Glasby and Tew, 2015, for an overview of mental health policy and practice). In response, campaigners have long called for a much greater focus on and investment in mental health services, and there has been growing public and media recognition of the importance of these issues (aided in part by a number of celebrities and public figures, including Prince Harry, speaking publicly about their own mental health). A stated aim of government has also been to create **parity of esteem** (ensuring that physical and mental health are given equal prominence). However, many argue that mental ill health is still poorly understood and the subject of stigma and fear; still misrepresented in the media; still a 'Cinderella service' within health and social care; and still massively under-funded (see **Key Sources 2**).

Key Sources 2: Struggling to achieve 'parity of esteem'

Mental health has long been regarded as a poor relation of the NHS. Years of under-investment mean that people with mental health problems often experience poorer access to services and lower quality of care than those with physical health conditions. For example, long waiting times are still common for psychological therapy; many people receive care in facilities outside of their home area because they cannot get the right care locally; and services for children and young people are widely regarded as inadequate.

In response to this, the Health and Social Care Act 2012 created a new legal responsibility for the NHS to deliver 'parity of esteem' between physical and mental health, which the coalition government subsequently committed to achieving by 2020. Parity of esteem means equal access to effective care and treatment; equal efforts to improve the quality of care; equal status within health care education and practice; equally high aspirations for service users; and equal status in the measurement of health outcomes (Royal College of Psychiatrists 2013) ...

The NHS has agreed an ambitious national strategy to improve mental health services in England, set out in The Five Year Forward View for Mental Health. To fund the strategy, the government indicated that £1 billion would be made available each year by 2020/21 (from money already earmarked for the NHS), and in July 2016 NHS England published an implementation plan indicating how this money would be phased in and, notionally, how it would be spent ...

[These commitments] build on ongoing work designed to put mental health on a more equal footing with physical health. One component of this is the new waiting time standards introduced for psychological therapies and for early intervention services for people experiencing a first episode of psychosis. This is the first time that access targets, which have been used in some parts of the NHS for many years, have been set for mental health, providing an important driver for improving access to these services ...

However, despite the increased profile of mental health at the national level, within local health systems much of this is overshadowed by concerns about funding ... An analysis conducted by The King's Fund found that in 2015/16, 40 per cent of mental health trusts in England received a real-terms decrease in their operating income. ... Workforce shortages in some areas of mental health care will also need to be addressed if parity is to become a reality. ...

Another important measure of parity is whether mental health receives sufficient focus within wider efforts to improve health care. There is good evidence that addressing mental and physical health needs together is better for patients and can be more cost-effective. On this front too there are concerns – for example, around the inclusion of mental health within STPs ... Although each STP is required to make reference to mental health, the degree of emphasis given to it varies, and there needs to be much greater focus on ensuring mental health care is integrated into other health and care services as part of these plans ...

The focus on parity of esteem is highly welcome ... However, there remains a sizeable gap between rhetoric and reality, particularly in relation to funding. Parity will not be achieved if mental health budgets remain vulnerable at times of financial pressure. To deliver the improvements set out in The Five Year Forward View for Mental Health, the next government will need to make sure that the money pledged reaches the front line. Otherwise parity will remain a distant goal.

Source: Extracted from: "Is there 'parity of esteem' between mental and physical health? big election questions", Chris Naylor, The King's Fund (blog), 19 May 2017. Full reference details and links to other sources can be found on The King's Fund website (www.kingsfund.org.uk).

Health v social care

In Chapter One, we reviewed the history of health and adult social care, commenting on the creation of a new National Health Service separate from local government-led adult social services. Although different structures have evolved in different parts of the UK, the health and social care divide remains a key fault line in our welfare state (and is also a common feature of other systems internationally – see **Facts and Figures 10**). Although it is now very dated, a strongly worded but helpful summary of the situation was provided by the Department of Health in a consultation that led to new legal powers for local health and social care systems to work together more creatively across agency boundaries. Although much has changed in the intervening years, this critique still feels very relevant:

> All too often when people have complex needs spanning both health and social care good quality services are sacrificed for sterile arguments about boundaries. When this happens people, often the most vulnerable in our society … and those who care for them find themselves in the no man's land between health and social services. This is not what people want or need. It places the needs of the organisation above the needs of the people they are there to serve. It is poor organisation, poor practice, poor use of taxpayers' money – it is unacceptable. (Department of Health, 1998, p 3)

This means that health and social care practitioners at local level can find themselves having to work with different agencies and professions, based in different organisations, with different cultures, policies, budgets, geographical boundaries, IT systems, legal frameworks and priorities. The potential for something to go wrong in this situation – for even one part of the jigsaw puzzle to get lost or fail to fit – is immense, and it is testimony to people's hard work and dedication that joint working across such complex fault lines happens to the extent that it does. Of course, when things go wrong or aren't joined-up, it can be extremely detrimental to the person concerned (as well as very frustrating, time consuming and difficult to put right for the different professionals).

A helpful way of thinking about this is to use a framework developed by Hudson and colleagues at the University of Leeds (see **Concepts and Debates 3**). This identifies a series of barriers to overcome when seeking to collaborate across the health and social care divide, as well as a series of principle for more effective partnership working.

Concepts and Debates 3: Barriers and enablers to partnership working

Key barriers	Structural (fragmentation of services across boundaries, complexity, lack of shared geographical boundaries)
	Procedural (different approaches to planning, IT, data sharing and accountability)
	Financial (different budgets, financial processes and ways of spending money)
	Professional/cultural (different values, competition between different professions, concerns about job security, different views about the role that users should play in their own care)
	Status and legitimacy (organisational tensions, and differences between elected and appointed leaders/agencies)
Enablers/ partnership principles	Acknowledging the need for partnership (recognising that health and social care are interdependent, and the extent to which we are building on a history of joint work)
	Clarity and realism of purpose (having a shared and realistic vision, together with some quick wins that can build confidence and win over sceptics)
	Commitment and ownership (leadership and organisational support)
	Development and maintenance of trust (difficult to achieve but helped by transparency, fairness and situations in which partners have a similar status, rather than a senior/junior partner)
	Clear and robust partnership arrangements (overcoming bureaucracy and complexity, being clear about the practicalities)
	Monitoring, review and organisational learning (reviewing from what's worked and learning/making changes accordingly)

Source: Hudson and Hardy (2002, p 54)

None of this is to underplay the importance of joint working across health and social care – no one would argue that we should work in isolation from each other or that we shouldn't link up and collaborate when this is in the best interests of the patient or will get a better outcome or will make better use of scarce resources. It's just that we're working in a system not designed with health and social care integration mind, and this can make joint working very difficult. As a famous article on the 'five laws of integration' put it (Leutz, 1999): 'you can't integrate a square peg and a round hole'.

Facts and Figures 10: Integrated care in the UK and beyond

Across the UK, there are a series of different policies and models that have emerged over time to try to deliver more integrated health and social care (Heenan and Birrell, 2018):

- In England, different governments have promoted pooled budgets between health and social care, integrated service provision, lead commissioning (where one partner takes a lead in commissioning services for a whole user group), integrated organisations, new joint funds to promote integration and interagency boards.
- In Scotland, we have seen joint health and social care strategies, the creation of new partnership bodies, the development of joint outcome indicators, managed clinical networks (to coordinate the efforts of clinicians across different parts of the system), and new integrated authorities to deliver joined-up care.
- In Wales, there have been Public Service Boards to coordinate care, a focus on public health and tackling health inequalities, and a new statutory framework for embedding partnership working and collaboration.
- In Northern Ireland, health and social services have been structurally integrated over many years, but additional initiatives include the creation of integration care partnerships to better promote integration at local level and overcome ongoing fragmentation.

Outside the UK, other interesting models include:

- US accountable care organisations, whereby a group of providers take joint responsibility for providing all of the care needed by a particular population, contracting with a commissioner to deliver particular outcomes and then negotiating how best to do this among themselves.
- Scandinavian health and social care (where community health and social care are often integrated at local council

> or municipality level, with hospital services provided at more of a regional level).
> • Community health centres in Ontario, with a strong focus on community development and meeting broader social, economic and environmental problems.
> • Healthy Kinzigtal population-based integrated systems in Germany.
> • A focus on 'one system, one budget' and on the importance of strong primary care in Canterbury, New Zealand.
> • The Nuka system of care in Alaska, seeking to integrate care for Alaska Native and American Indian people and seeing the community as owners (rather than recipients) of health services, with a role in service design.
> • Jönköping County Council in Sweden, seeking to integrate care around the needs of Esther, a fictitious older person, and developing a 'Passion for Life' programme (with older people meeting in community settings for 'life cafes' to explore how to improve health and well-being).

For all that integrating health and social is a key priority in many different systems, it is interesting that no system has been able to identify a full solution (including in Northern Ireland, where the two sectors are structurally integrated). As discussed in Chapter One, Powell (2018) also identified the integration of health and social as a longstanding goal that has been pursued throughout the history of the NHS – but with success so far elusive. While there is lots we can do to provide more coordinated care to people with complex and multiple needs, perhaps the lessons here are that very big organisations/systems will always have boundaries, and that we may always need to find ways to work across such boundaries where this is in the interest of the people using our services. Ultimately, real life is usually more complex and messier than the structures and systems we create in our legal frameworks, our welfare organisations, our services and our professional training.

Medical cure v public health/prevention

In Chapter One, we saw how the NHS has tended to focus on medical cure, and how health and social services have sometimes been better at providing support in a crisis rather than keeping people healthy and well in the first place (see also Chapter Four for discussion of health and well-being). The latter has been the responsibility of public health (which, at different times, has been based within the NHS or local government).

According to the World Health Organization (WHO):

> Public Health is defined as "the art and science of preventing disease, prolonging life and promoting health through the organized efforts of society" ... Activities to strengthen public health capacities and service aim to provide conditions under which people can maintain to be healthy, improve their health and wellbeing, or prevent the deterioration of their health. Public health focuses on the entire spectrum of health and wellbeing, not only the eradication of particular diseases. Many activities are targeted at populations such as health campaigns. Public health services also include the provision of personal services to individual persons, such as vaccinations, behavioural counselling, or health advice. (www.euro.who.int/en/health-topics/Health-systems/public-health-services)

This is crucial work, but – a little like the discussion of mental health and **parity of esteem** – has tended to be less valued and less well funded than services focusing on medical cure (particularly hospital services). In England, the transfer of public health from the NHS to local government in 2012 brought lots of opportunities for public health to work alongside broader services (such as education, planning and economic development), but has also led to widespread cuts (given the nature of current local government finances).

In addition to the skills and experience of public health experts, many health and adult social services have been trying to develop more preventative approaches – continuing to meet the needs of people in a crisis, but also seeking to keep as many people as possible healthy and well so that they don't experience a crisis or need formal services in the first place. For example, in adult social care, many councils are trying to improve the advice and signposting they provide when someone first gets in touch (so that people with low-level needs get meaningful information about where to go for support, even if they don't meet the council's eligibility criteria). Where people do need formal support, councils have often developed their home care services on the basis of a **reablement** approach (see **Key Sources 3**), so that people receive a short, intensive period of support to see if they can return to independence and not need ongoing services. In both health and social care, **intermediate care** services seek to support people (often older people) at risk of hospital admission or after they come out of hospital, either via rapid response nursing support in the home, or via a short, rehabilitative stay in an intermediate care unit (with a view to supporting the person to return home as quickly as possible).

Key Sources 3: Reablement 'at a glance'

The focus of reablement is on restoring independent functioning rather than resolving health care issues. The objective is to help people relearn how to do things for themselves rather than the conventional home care approach of doing things for people. Reablement appears to be welcomed by people receiving the service, and represents an investment that may produce savings.

Research on reablement has examined whether it is a better approach to supporting people than conventional home care. Key questions are whether better outcomes can be achieved, and for whom, and whether savings can be made through investment in reablement. Findings are broadly positive. People using reablement experience greater improvements in physical functioning, health-related quality of life and social care outcomes compared with people using standard home care ...

Reablement services are for people with disabilities and those who are frail or recovering from an illness or injury. The aim is to help people regain the ability to perform their usual activities, like cooking meals, washing and getting about, so they can do things for themselves again, stay independent and live in their own home ... Reablement is usually non-chargeable for the first six weeks, which means it is free of charge even for people who usually pay for all or part of their care.

If a person is referred to a reablement service, reablement workers will visit them in their home, assess their abilities and needs and agree goals. Over the next few days or weeks the individual will be supported to regain physical function, relearn skills and if necessary learn different ways of doing daily tasks such as meal preparation, washing and dressing ...

Reablement services are run by local authorities, so eligibility can vary depending on where you live. They tend to be targeted at those for whom reablement will be most likely to lead to improvement. This means prioritising those people who are most likely to benefit by regaining physical function and improving their independence.

For this reason, in some areas, people with certain conditions such as dementia, or those who are near the end of their life, tend not to be offered reablement. In other areas, these groups may be offered reablement services, depending on their individual circumstances. Ideally people should be referred for reablement because of their needs and not their medical diagnoses.

Source: *At a glance 54: Reablement: a guide for families and carers*, SCIE, www.scie.org.uk/publications/ataglance/ataglance54.asp

In practice, health and social care have found it difficult to develop preventative approaches over the long-term and in ways which become core to mainstream services. As a result, many preventative projects are organised on the basis of small scale or time-limited pilots, and it has been difficult to genuinely re-balance the whole health and social care system so that prevention is at its heart. This is for a number of inter-connected reasons:

- Services have to prioritise people in crisis or severe need, so freeing up resources to also focus on prevention is challenging.
- It is hard to prove that a new project or service has actually prevented something from happening, so generating a convincing evidence base is difficult.
- Working with someone to help them help themselves often takes longer and requires different skills to doing something for someone.
- There has been concern that some preventative services have tended (not unreasonably) to work with people most likely to benefit from this approach – but this leaves unanswered questions about what happens to everyone else. A good example is older people with dementia, who have sometimes been excluded from reablement projects. This leads to accusations that pilots are 'cherry-picking' the people with whom they will work.
- Embedding prevention would probably need significant and sustained cultural change across all our services – and this is hard to achieve.
- Media and political timescales often require immediate results, and preventative approaches (even if successful) might take many years to bear fruit.

For all these reasons, prevention is a key feature of many policy documents, but remains challenging to achieve at sufficient scale in practice.

Managing service pressures and reconfigurations

At the time of writing, the financial challenges described in Chapter Two are leading to a series of difficult and often controversial decisions about the best way to organise services (and even about whether some services should be provided at all). In England, for example, many hospital services are responding to the current financial context by seeking to merge, thereby creating very large organisations with multiple hospitals, large budgets, lots of staff and (hopefully) greater scope to achieve economies of scale and savings targets. Time will tell whether this is a successful tactic, or whether it merely distracts attention from the challenges of frontline service provision and creates organisations that are too big to manage effectively. Different areas of the country are also experimenting with new models of health and care, seeking to integrate their hospital and community/primary care services and/or their health and social care services in response to rapidly rising need and demand. Some **Clinical Commissioning Groups** are also seeking to reduce funding for (or change access to) IVF, access to non-urgent surgery for people who continue to smoke or who are struggling to lose weight, and hip/knee surgery for people experiencing lower levels of pain. Typically, this is not why people came to work in the NHS, and the current context is proving extremely challenging (see Chapter Six for a discussion of job satisfaction and stress). Ironically, this is something that colleagues in adult social are well used to, since they have long assessed people in need against a set of increasingly stringent eligibility criteria. However, the fact remains that both health and social care are under significant pressure – and the realities of delivering care form the next section of this book.

Further resources

Helpful discussions of **NHS reorganisations** are provided by Edwards (2010) and Walshe (2003). The former is available to download free of charge from the NHS Confederation.

There have been various calls for greater **NHS independence** over time, including by Glasby et al (2007). Peckham et al (2005) review arguments around **decentralisation, centralisation and devolution** in publicly funded health services, exploring the implications for the English NHS.

NHS Improvement provides practical resources for commissioners and providers seeking to shift **care closer to home** (https://improvement.nhs.uk/resources/moving-healthcare-closer-home/), while the former NHS Institute for Improvement and Innovation published an online review of the evidence and key lessons when seeking to shift care (www.birmingham.ac.uk/Documents/college-social-sciences/social policy/HSMC/publications/2007/Getting-the-basics-right.pdf).

Key priorities for **mental health** services are set out in *The Five Year Forward View for Mental Health* (NHS England/Mental Health Taskforce, 2016), and an introductory textbook is provided by Glasby and Tew (2015).

For a guide to **integrated care** in the four counties of the UK, see:

- Heenan and Birrell's (2018) introductory textbook
- The King's Fund's (Ham et al, 2013) guide to *Integrated Care in Northern Ireland, Scotland and Wales*

Useful journals (with lots of articles from research, policy and practice) include:

- *Journal of Integrated Care*
- *International Journal of Integrated Care*

Introductions to **public health** are published by Hunter et al (2010) and Baggott (2011, 2013). The Faculty of Public Health (www.fph.org.uk) is the standard setting body for specialists in public health in the UK.

The Social Care Institute for Excellence (SCIE) produces a series of free resources on **reablement** (www.scie.org.uk/reablement), while Allen and Glasby (2010) set out 'ten high impact changes' when seeking to embed **prevention** in health and social care. Allen et al (2013) explore how councils decide how to invest in prevention and what they think works for older people.

Part 2:

People and practice

4

The social context of health and social care

Working in health and social care means working with people –
often at crucial times in their lives and when they are at their most
vulnerable and distressed. At a very basic level, this means that we
have to understand people and their families, their communities and
the way in which our society works in order to be able to deliver high
quality care and make sense of our work. This is true in all kinds of
different ways, but the current chapter focuses on a small number
of key concepts and frameworks to help illustrate the importance of
the social context in which we deliver care. These include:

- Health, well-being and independence
- Health inequalities and the social determinants of health
- Social divisions and social construction
- Empowerment and user involvement

Health, well-being and independence

In many ways, it is major irony that our NHS is not really a 'health
service' at all – but more of a 'sickness service'. Lots of health services
involve operating on people, giving medication to cure a disease or
treat symptoms, and working with people to help them recover after
an illness, an accident or an operation. These are potentially life-
saving interventions, and many of them feel miraculous, at the very
edge of science. Anyone watching the BBC documentary *Surgeons*,

for example, can see what difference major surgery makes to people's lives, how complex the operations featured are, and what astounding technical skills are required. Most of us could never cut into a fellow human being, open up their chest and heart, and stitch them back together afterwards – either emotionally or in terms of technical knowledge and ability – and we're rightly in awe of people who can. However, although health is often interpreted as the absence of disease, this is quite a negative definition (it is defined by what it isn't: someone is healthy if they are not ill). In contrast, a number of approaches focus more on positive health, defined by the WHO from 1948 onwards as 'a state of complete physical, mental and social well-being and not merely the absence of disease or infirmity' (www. who.int/about/mission/en/). Crucially, this definition includes both physical and mental health – and the latter is an interesting example of these issues. While most of our health and social services focus on 'mental illness' (a negative, disease-orientated approach which might only apply to those we define as being unwell), it is also possible to think about what we do in terms of 'mental health' or 'mental well-being,' more positive concepts that apply to all of us. As Glasby and Tew (2015, p 4) have argued:

> Positive mental health includes the ability to understand and make sense of our surroundings, to cope with change and to connect with other people. When mentally well, we are aware of and have control over different strands of our life, we have the will to live life to its full potential; things make sense to us.

While these debates might feel fairly far removed from the realities of frontline services, the definitions we adopt matter and can influence how we shape policy and practice. Curing someone when they are ill or injured is different from supporting someone to stay healthy in the first place, and it might need different skills and approaches. Moreover, creating happy and healthy communities and making sure that people have the relationships and resources to live a good life might benefit many more people in one go than intervening in an emergency when one person has a serious illness or accident.

Linked to notions of health is the concept of 'well-being' (and this is mentioned directly in the WHO mission set out above). This is difficult to define, but different schools of thought often focus on the extent to which people's needs are met (including social and psychological needs) and/or the extent to which we flourish as human beings and are reaching our potential. In England, the local bodies responsible for bringing together the NHS and local government to plan joint responses to need are known as **Health and Wellbeing Boards**, with responsibility for producing a joint assessment of the needs of the local area, developing a joint strategy to meet these needs and improving the integration of health and social care. From 2014, the **Care Act** consolidated lots of previous adult social care legislation which had grown up piecemeal since 1948, and sought to re-orientate services towards a greater focus on promoting individual well-being (see **Key Sources 4** for Care Act definitions). While this was widely welcomed, the reality at ground level has felt little different to date, with severe financial pressures in local government making it difficult to do anything other than the bare minimum. However, having this Act on the statute books still feels an important statement of intent, and it remains the law – even if many areas are struggling to implement their new duties in practice.

Key Sources 4: Section 1 of the Care Act 2014

1. Promoting individual well-being

  (1) The general duty of a local authority, in exercising a function under this Part in the case of an individual, is to promote that individual's well-being.

  (2) "Well-being", in relation to an individual, means that individual's well-being so far as relating to any of the following—

    (a) personal dignity (including treatment of the individual with respect);

    (b) physical and mental health and emotional well-being;

(c) protection from abuse and neglect;

(d) control by the individual over day-to-day life (including over care and support, or support, provided to the individual and the way in which it is provided);

(e) participation in work, education, training or recreation;

(f) social and economic well-being;

(g) domestic, family and personal relationships;

(h) suitability of living accommodation;

(i) the individual's contribution to society.

(3) In exercising a function under this Part in the case of an individual, a local authority must have regard to the following matters in particular—

(a) the importance of beginning with the assumption that the individual is best-placed to judge the individual's well-being;

(b) the individual's views, wishes, feelings and beliefs;

(c) the importance of preventing or delaying the development of needs for care and support or needs for support and the importance of reducing needs of either kind that already exist;

(d) the need to ensure that decisions about the individual are made having regard to all the individual's circumstances (and are not based only on the individual's age or appearance or any condition of the individual's or aspect of the individual's behaviour which might lead others to make unjustified assumptions about the individual's well-being);

(e) the importance of the individual participating as fully as possible in decisions relating to the exercise of the function concerned and being provided with the information and support necessary to enable the individual to participate;

> (f)   the importance of achieving a balance between
>   the individual's well-being and that of any friends
>   or relatives who are involved in caring for the
>   individual;
> (g)   the need to protect people from abuse and
>   neglect;
> (h)   the need to ensure that any restriction on the
>   individual's rights or freedom of action that
>   is involved in the exercise of the function is
>   kept to the minimum necessary for achieving
>   the purpose for which the function is being
>   exercised.
>
> Source: Original text of the Care Act 2014, available via www.legislation.
> gov.uk

For adult social care in particular, another key term is 'independence' – even if people are ill, frail or disabled, they can still be independent. However, this is often mistakenly taken to mean that people are able to do everything for themselves – and this can be misleading. In practice, none of us do everything for ourselves, and we're all interdependent on others to meet some of our needs. Life would be very lonely indeed if we were all fully independent from each other (a little like Robinson Crusoe on his island before he meets Man Friday). Instead, disabled people's organisations have stressed the importance of **independent living** – which they define as having choice and control over one's life. This is discussed in more detail in Chapter Two and is central to much recent adult social policy. Even if some people need some practical assistance with aspects of their daily living, they can still exercise just as much choice and control over their lives as anyone else (unless services and broader society deny people this).

Linked to positive notions of health and to concepts of independent living is the concept of **assets-based approaches** to health and social care. Many of our current services are 'deficit-based' – they exist to identify what is 'wrong' with someone and then try to put it right. This can be exactly what's needed in many situations (if I have cancer, I need someone to help diagnose what's wrong and try to cure me). However, for other things, it can be a very negative way of working (both for staff and for people using services) – encouraging people to emphasise what they can't do for themselves rather than focusing on what they can do. This has been a key debate in adult social care, with a number of service models which seek to start from what people can already do for themselves, what makes a good life for them, the networks and supports that people rely on in their everyday life in their local community, and so on. This is very different to the care management model that dominated adult social care in the 1990s and 2000s, which sought to assess people's needs and determine whether they were eligible for support (against increasingly tight eligibility criteria). In practice, this forces people to stress how dependent and in need they are, and to minimise any natural supports. The consequences of this are set out in **Voices of Experience 6** while **Concepts and Debates 4** summarises the principles and implications of more assets–based approaches.

Voices of Experience 6: The problem of focusing on deficits

"Social care is facing tough times. Social workers are deployed principally as border patrol, policing access to increasingly insufficient resources against a growing clamour of seemingly limitless need. The only access point, a humiliating demonstration of vulnerability and dependency. It is a deficit model that has dominated practice and policy for decades. Yet it is now clearer than ever before that it is unsustainable ..." (Paul Burstow MP – subsequently architect of the 2014 Care Act)

"Current social care law... is set up to focus exclusively on eligible needs and how services alone can meet these needs. Assessments are designed to 'gate-keep' services and can require people to go through a demeaning and disempowering process focused entirely on proving their vulnerability, often only to find they are deemed ineligible. Support which is or could be offered by family carers

*and others is often invisible in the current system, with any needs
which are currently being met by carers treated as non-existent."
(Alex Fox, Chief Executive, Shared Lives)*

*"Increasingly, within local government, there is a recognition
that we are approaching a moment of crisis. Both short-term and
long-term pressures on public services... mean that we need to
think hard not simply about how we deliver our current services,
but fundamentally about what a council is and what it does (and
does not do), about the nature of public service and about the
boundaries between citizens, state and communities." (Jonathan
Carr-West, Local Government Information Unit)*

Source: all quotes from Glasby et al's (2013) policy paper on new
approaches to adult social care: '*Turning the Welfare State Upside
Down?': Developing a new adult social care offer*, www.birmingham.ac.uk/
Documents/college-social-sciences/social-policy/HSMC/publications/
PolicyPapers/policy-paper-fifteen.pdf

Concepts and Debates 4: Assets-based approaches

*There are many examples of excellent asset-based approaches,
and a growing body of evidence of their impact... Common
examples include:*

- *local area coordination (LAC)*
- *Shared Lives schemes*
- *community circles*
- *community enterprise development*
- *asset-based community development (ABCD)*
- *time banks*
- *peer support*
- *community navigators*
- *social prescribing*

*In many cases, these examples are small scale, impacting on
too few people. More could be done to support asset-based*

approaches to become more mainstream, while ensuring they remain community-based and community-led. (SCIE, 2017, p 2)

What would a local health and care system look like were we able to create asset-based areas and scale up the most promising innovations? Such a system, in our view, would have the following features:

- *People's health, care and support shaped through strength-based conversations that seek to address a whole person's life, rather just assessing a narrow set of needs*
- *Services are co-produced with the people whose lives they touch. This means that everyone involved identifies priorities, co-designs services and systems and works together wherever possible to co-deliver the work that takes place*
- *A flourishing range of community assets and peer networks focused on building the knowledge, skills and confidence of people to self-manage their care*
- *Neighbourhood-based multidisciplinary and integrated teams, working with communities and volunteers and focusing on what is important to each person. This can be done through personalised planning which aims to include all aspects of family and community life*
- *Budgets are devolved as far as possible down to neighbourhoods, families and individuals, maximising choice and control over how money is spent on people's care*
- *Community buildings, including care homes and primary care centres, are reassigned as multi-use community resources*
- *Services are funded and measured on the basis that they make positive changes in people's lives, in terms of wellbeing, resilience, independence, connections to others and the ability to self-care*
- *A thriving and sustainable voluntary, community and social enterprise sector, working alongside people, families, communities and the health and care system. (SCIE, 2018, p 3)*

Health inequalities and the social determinants of health

While many health and social services focus on individual biology or on an individual's ability to carry out activities of daily living, people's needs are heavily influenced by the lifestyle they have led, the community and society in which they live, the resources they possess and the relationships they have with others. As the WHO explains:

> The social determinants of health are the conditions in which people are born, grow, live, work and age. These circumstances are shaped by the distribution of money, power and resources at global, national and local levels. The social determinants of health are mostly responsible for health inequities – the unfair and avoidable differences in health status seen within and between countries. (www.who.int/social_determinants/ sdh_definition/en/)

In England, the Marmot Review (2010, p 3) into **health inequalities** observes:

> People with higher socioeconomic position in society have a greater array of life chances and more opportunities to lead a flourishing life. They also have better health. The two are linked: the more favoured people are, socially and economically, the better their health. This link between social conditions and health is not a footnote to the 'real' concerns with health – health care and unhealthy behaviours – it should become the main focus. Consider one measure of social position: education. People with university degrees have better health and longer lives than those without. For people aged 30 and above, if everyone without a degree had their death rate reduced to that of people with degrees, there would be 202,000 fewer premature deaths each year. Surely this is a goal worth striving for.
>
> It is the view of all of us associated with this Review that we could go a long way to achieving that remarkable improvement by giving more people the life chances currently enjoyed by

the few. The benefits of such efforts would be wider than lives saved. People in society would be better off in many ways: in the circumstances in which they are born, grow, live, work, and age. People would see improved well-being, better mental health and less disability, their children would flourish, and they would live in sustainable, cohesive communities.

While the UK does well when the quality of its health services is compared internationally (see Chapter One), it experiences widespread **health inequalities** (differences in health depending on one's social position). In such an unequal society, our health services can only do so much by themselves to keep us well and to help us recover when we're sick. If we want even better health, then we may need to think differently about the broader society within which we live and the role of other services and sectors (such as education, employment, community development and so on). To tackle health inequalities, the Marmot Review called for action against six policy objectives, some of which may involve health and social care, but many of which are much broader (**Key Sources 5**).

Key Sources 5: Tackling health inequalities and the social determinants of health

In England, the Marmot Review (2010) concluded that tackling health inequalities would require concerted action against six policy objectives:

1. Give every child the best start in life
2. Enable all children, young people and adults to maximise their capabilities and have control over their lives
3. Create fair employment and good work for all
4. Ensure healthy standard of living for all
5. Create and develop healthy and sustainable places and communities
6. Strengthen the role and impact of ill health prevention

In the words of the Review (p 16):

Inequalities are a matter of life and death, of health and sickness, of well-being and misery. The fact that in England today people in different social circumstances experience avoidable differences in health, well-being and length of life is, quite simply, unfair. Creating a fairer society is fundamental to improving the health of the whole population and ensuring a fairer distribution of good health.

Inequalities in health arise because of inequalities in society – in the conditions in which people are born, grow, live, work, and age. So close is the link between particular social and economic features of society and the distribution of health among the population, that the magnitude of health inequalities is a good marker of progress towards creating a fairer society. Taking action to reduce inequalities in health does not require a separate health agenda, but action across the whole of society.

Internationally, the WHO Commission on Social Determinants of Health (WHO, 2008, executive summary) calls for action to close this health gap within a generation:

Our children have dramatically different life chances depending on where they were born. In Japan or Sweden they can expect to live more than 80 years; in Brazil, 72 years; India, 63 years; and in one of several African countries, fewer than 50 years. And within countries, the differences in life chances are dramatic and are seen worldwide. The poorest of the poor have high levels of illness and premature mortality. But poor health is not confined to those worst off. In countries at all levels of income, health and illness follow a social gradient: the lower the socioeconomic position, the worse the health. It does not have to be this way and it is not right that it should be like this. Where systematic differences in health are judged to be avoidable by reasonable action they are, quite simply, unfair. It is this that we label health inequity. Putting right these inequities – the huge and remediable differences in health between and within countries – is a matter of social justice. Reducing health inequities is, for the Commission on Social Determinants of Health (hereafter, the Commission), an ethical imperative. Social injustice is killing people on a grand scale.

Social divisions and social construction

One of the ways in which we make sense of a complicated world is to divide people into groups, and to make working assumptions about how someone might behave based on the group to which we have allocated them. These are inevitably vast over-simplifications, but they can be a helpful shorthand for understanding what's going on around us and how to navigate the world. For example, we might divide people into male and female. If we assume that some men can find it difficult to talk about their feelings, we might reflect that they could be less willing to seek help for a mental health problem or, in extreme cases, more at risk of suicide. We might conclude that some men seem more prone to violence and aggression than women, and that men with severe mental health problems might be more likely to be violent to others than women. Equally, it is often assumed that some women might take their distress out on themselves (for example, through self-harm) or indirectly (for example, through starting a fire) rather than through direct aggression.

These examples immediately illustrate the importance but also the dangers of such an approach. It can certainly be helpful to be mindful of the potential situations above (for example, checking out if a man is in distress, but struggling to admit it). However, it would also be very easy to make a series of misunderstandings and mistakes (failing to check as carefully if a woman is in distress; assuming a man might be violent and accidentally creating something of a self-fulfilling prophecy; failing to consider male self-harm because we wrongly assume that distress might be taken out on others, and so on). Having a working hypothesis about the world and what may be going on is useful; allowing this to tip over into stereotypes and working solely on the basis of assumptions is dangerous.

Another consequence of our tendency to put people in groups is that this process is seldom neutral or value-free. Whether we realise it or not, we tend to organise our society in a way which means that some groups of people have more access to power and resources than others. We refer to these as **social divisions**, and we know that people's experiences, opportunities, identities and life chances are all influenced by whether we are upper, middle or working class; male or female; black or white; gay or straight; young or old; disabled or non-disabled, and so on. Usually, this involves making assumptions about groups of people and, when we fail to challenge these assumptions, discriminating against particular groups. For example, it was once assumed that pretty much everyone was part of a heterosexual family, with two parents and kids, a male breadwinner and a female head of the household who would cook, clean and look after the children and possibly any older relatives. Indeed, my great-grandmother worked at the Cadbury factory in Birmingham and had to leave work when she got married, as her employer simply assumed that all women would give up work to concentrate on their husband, their home and a new family. While things feel very different now, we still have situations where senior positions in many fields are dominated by men, where men are often paid more than women and where women may take on more responsibility than men for household and caring responsibilities. Moreover, these legacies and assumptions are still hard-wired into our health and social services. Despite changes over time, professions such as nursing and roles such as home carer or care assistant are still predominantly female occupations, as deep down these are considered to be 'women's work'. Certainly, I remember working as a care assistant in a number of care homes, and people (staff and service users) being surprised and often a little confused that there was a male carer on shift.

A really interesting element of all this is our tendency to assume that the social divisions described above are biological and inevitable – when often they are social in origin. While there are biological differences between men and women, the assumptions about 'women's work' referred to above aren't biological – they are to do with the different roles, values and behaviours that we associate with men and women. We therefore distinguish between 'sex' (biological differences) and 'gender' (assumptions about male and female roles). Similarly, we often assume that race is biological, when really there are more biological differences between people of the same race. Instead, race is social (assumptions we make about people based on their skin colour) – and most commentators now put this word in inverted commas ('race') to convey the fact that it might be in everyday usage, but doesn't really exist as a biological concept. We also see same similar issues in debates about ageing. Although we use phrases like 'the elderly', older age isn't really a biological category (there are some very frail young people and incredibly fit and healthy 90-year-olds). It's more that our society assumes that people will leave work at around 65 (these assumptions are now being questioned as a result of an ageing population and financial pressures on pensions) – and 'elderly people' will often behave in a particular way. There is simply no one point at which we stop being 'young' or 'middle-aged' and become 'elderly' – these are just categories and labels that we've created to help make sense of the world, but have then forgotten that these are just artificial constructs. In recognition of this, some people try to talk about 'older people' rather than 'the elderly'.

We refer to this as **social construction** – a tendency to assume that something is natural, biological and inevitable, when actually it's an artificial category that we have created ourselves and (often unwittingly) embedded in the way we organise our society. Perhaps the best example of this is the debate about **independent living** described above. For many years, our health and social services saw disability as a biological category (there were some people who had something wrong with their bodies, and medical science could either cure them/help them recover, or sometimes it couldn't – in which case people would need 'care' to do the things they couldn't do for themselves). In one sense this is utter nonsense – advances in science mean that we now know that all of us have something wrong with our bodies in one way or another (there's no such thing as biological and genetic perfection, so in one sense we're all flawed). However, it was disabled people themselves, drawing inspiration from civil rights campaigns around 'race' and gender, who challenged this situation and pioneered alternatives ways of thinking. For them, some people had 'impairments' (biological limitations or physical/mental health problems) – but the main issue was disability (which they described as the way in which society discriminates against people with impairments). This is known as a **social model of disability**, and it was revolutionary (to me, it's the single most revolutionary idea I've come across in all my work and it has fundamentally changed what I do, how I do it and how I see the world).

Thus, if someone is in a wheelchair and can't reach a light switch we could argue that the problem is individual and biological (the person has a physical impairment, and a solution might be to intervene medically – a **medical model of disability**). However, we could also argue that the problem is socially constructed – the main issue arises not because of the person's impairment, but because we locate our light switches at a height which is comfortable for an adult standing up. Here the problem could be solved not by operating on the individual, but by simply moving the light switch (or inventing another way of operating the lights which doesn't need a switch at all). Interestingly, this one intervention (changing the built environment) would be much cheaper than individual medical cures, would work well for all people using wheelchairs (not just an individual person we've operated on), and could also work for other groups of people (such as children). Until a disabled person pointed this out to us, we probably never even thought about it – we just 'naturally' put the light switch at standing height, and never considered the thought processes and assumptions that went behind this decision. We then built this in to how we do things, so that the vast majority of light switches are automatically put at this height in the vast majority of buildings, thus systematically (but completely unwittingly) making things harder for and discriminating against a whole group of people. When we take a step back, we probably do this in all kinds of ways (see **Voices of Experience 7** for examples), and our lives, our attitudes and our health and social services are all heavily influenced by social divisions, social constructions and assumptions about what is 'normal'.

Voices of Experience 7: Designing services from dominant perspectives

While we often believe that we are treating everyone the same, this can easily mean discriminating against particular groups if we fail to recognise that many of our services are designed on the basis of assumptions about who a 'typical' service user might be or what they might need. Below are examples from my experience training as a social worker:

- When I worked as a care assistant in a care home, the kitchen staff used to assume that everyone would like a 'traditional' roast dinner at the weekend, without necessarily recognising that what is 'traditional' may depend on people's backgrounds. This didn't work well for an older Asian woman, a Chinese woman or a vegetarian from a White UK background, as these people were used to eating different things before they entered the care home and there were no alternatives provided. This never occurred to the kitchen staff, who were trying to be kind and to provide a treat for residents.
- A health clinic held on a Friday afternoon in a predominantly Muslim area of the city clashed with Friday prayers – and staff were perplexed when very few people came along.

- When I was training, disability benefits for people of working age had a care component and a mobility component. Attendance Allowance (for disabled people aged 65 or over) only had a care component (it was implicitly assumed that older people don't go out much so don't need a mobility component).

- Care home funding for services for people with learning difficulties or people with physical impairments of working age tended to be much higher than funding for older people with similar needs, as it was assumed that younger people would need to do things outside the home during the day, while older people would stay in the care home 24/7 and therefore need less funding.

- A lot of carers' support was targeted at people carrying out physical care tasks on behalf of someone with a physical impairment, forgetting that caring for someone with a mental health problem may be different. Most support was also based on the idea of families living near each other, without thinking about people caring at a distance.

- Lots of carers from black and ethnic minority communities weren't asked whether they needed support, as some workers assumed that people from these communities 'look after their own' and would not want support.

Arising out of this discussion, there are two final points to add:

1. *Multiple identities:* lots of attempts to overcome discrimination focus on single aspects of people's identities (tackling sex discrimination, racial discrimination, disability discrimination, and so on). However, all of us have multiple identities, and these inevitably shape our experiences. Thus, a disabled man may have a different experience to a disabled women; a young working-class black person may have different experiences to an older upper-class black person, and so on. Even when we're trying not to make assumptions about people, we can fall into the trap of making new assumptions by simply seeing them through one lens.

This was pointed out to me by a disabled friend after I'd found funding to install a disabled toilet in the place where I worked (it was a very old building in a conservation area, so getting the necessary building works agreed and funded was tricky). I felt good about myself – but my friend pointed out that having a male toilet, a female toilet and a disabled toilet implied that she was disabled first and foremost before she was a woman, and that the way we build accessible toilets assumes that a disabled man may have more in common with a disabled women than with other men or women respectively. I still don't know the answer to this, and having the new toilet seemed better than not having it – but I can't help feeling that she was right.

2. *Equality of inputs v equality of outcomes*: while adult social care is often restricted to people with very significant needs and low incomes, the NHS prides itself on its commitment to treating everybody the same, irrespective of their means. These are important and attractive principles, but arguably mask a number of dilemmas. 'Treating everyone the same' can mean ensuring that the same services are provided everywhere, or could mean different areas of the country with different needs offering different services to try to achieve the same outcomes for local people. If people start off unequal, then treating everyone the same can only ever perpetuate existing inequalities (and could even make these worse if we inadvertently design care from a 'white UK' perspective and end up treating some groups less favourably as a result). When it comes to issues such as 'race', this can lead to a 'colour-blind' approach, where our desire to treat everyone equally can lead to us failing to take sufficient account of social divisions, disadvantage and discrimination. Perhaps we too often focus on 'equality of input' (giving everyone the same) rather than 'equality of outcome' (treating different people differently to try to achieve the same overall outcomes for everyone)?

Empowerment and user involvement

In Chapter One, we saw how the NHS has long been dominated by the medical profession, and how adult social care emerged out of case workers assessing people to see who was 'deserving' of assistance. Post-war society was arguably much more deferential than now, and there was a strong assumption that 'doctor knows best'. Services were therefore planned and delivered by welfare professionals, who were seen as experts and whose decisions we would do well to follow. The term 'patient' is a really interesting one in this respect, as it implies a very passive role, simply waiting quietly for the professional to 'do their thing'. Over time, however, social attitudes have changed, and many people now want and expect to have much greater say about what care they receive and how it is delivered. Doctors and other professionals are still experts, but we are also experts in our own lives and often have a strong sense of what works well for us (given our situations, networks and communities), what a good outcome would look like and how we might want to be treated. This might be particularly true for people who have an ongoing or life-long condition, as they will have acquired significant experience of living with that condition, and may know as much about many aspects of it as the professionals with whom they're working. Current services are therefore seen as much more of a partnership of equals, where the practitioner and the person using services each bring something unique and distinctive to the encounter, and where what works well for one person may not be such a good outcome for someone else. These changes are partly reflected in the growing recognition of the importance of **assets-based approaches** (see **Concepts and Debates 4**), but have also led to a shift in the culture of some of our health and social services, and to a greater emphasis on concepts such as **user involvement** and **empowerment**:

1. It is now broadly accepted that people using health and social care have a right to be involved in decisions about their own care and treatment, and sometimes in decisions about how services are

designed and delivered more generally. This might be because of a number of inter-linked factors and rationales:

- These are publicly funded services which, in one sense, belong to all of us – so we have a democratic right to be involved.
- These services are so important to our well-being – it's really important to us that we have a say.
- Some things work well for one person, but wouldn't work as well for another – so we need to find out what's important to the person and how services can help deliver a good outcome for them.
- Choice and control can be beneficial in themselves – we tend to feel better and do better in situations where we can influence what happens to us.
- People using services and their families have crucial expertise which can help us improve individual care and services as a whole.

2. It is fairly broadly accepted (but perhaps not always) that there is a power imbalance between people providing health and social care, and people using these services. In some situations, this imbalance can be very stark – for example, when a person with mental health problems is being taken into hospital against their will; when the state decides that a parent is not capable of continuing to care for their own child; or when we're really ill and distressed and don't have the same degree of confidence or capability that we would normally possess. In one sense, the state and its employees decide what services are provided, how they are delivered and who gets what – and we're often expected to be grateful for this (despite the fact that they are services which are funded by all of us and belong to all of us for the collective good). In recognition of this, anything that helps to break down potential barriers between the professional and the service user, and to share power, is probably a good thing – creating more equal relationships and enabling people to take much greater control of their condition and their lives. This is discussed in further detail in Chapter Two around the **personalisation agenda** – a particularly strong form of

sharing power and building on the expertise of the individual and those around them.

Arising out of the debates, there are lots of practical mechanisms for people using health and social services to feed back their experience of receiving care, contribute to discussions about future service delivery and even to become more formally involved. In social work education, for example, people with experience of using services and carers might both be involved in selecting students for social work programmes, teaching and assessing work, as well as being part of recruitment processes as students qualify and seek their first roles. The same is also true in many areas of health and social care research, where service users and carers may well be involved in a number of studies as 'co-researchers', helping to design the research, gather and analyse data, and disseminate findings. Much of this has been captured in a key slogan which is now common in health and social care: 'nothing about me without me'.

While there are lots of accounts of empowerment and involvement, a famous and longstanding approach is set out by Arnstein (1969) in her 'ladder of participation'. This sets out different degrees of involvement (portrayed as a ladder) from non-participation to tokenistic approaches (simply informing people of what you're doing, consulting people on changes that are happening anyway, or seeking people's views simply to placate them and without really listening) through to situations where the citizen genuinely controls what happens. This is particularly helpful, as it starts to identify the extent of power sharing, and also reveals some of the less positive aspects of these debates. While services know that they're meant to be involving people, and while they can probably see some benefits to this, it can be difficult for people who are used to being in control of a situation letting go and genuinely engaging with others about what might work better in future. At the very least, this can be time consuming and difficult to do well. It can also be very messy and complicated – it's usually much quicker and easier to decide something yourself than it is to discuss with a range of other people, who might have different perspectives and not agree. In a worst case scenario, we might even resent other people being involved in decisions which we see as ours to take, genuinely believing that we know best and jealously holding on to power. On other occasions, we might really want to involve people using services in the decisions we're taking, but the politics of the situation might mean that we have a little real choice and we don't want to set people up to fail by asking them about something that we know is likely to happen anyway. In these situations, so-called 'involvement' can become tokenistic or even cynical – being seen to ask people what they think, but not really being interested in or trying to act on the answers they give us. In some situations, managers or practitioners can even 'play the user card' – seeking to gather views that support their pre-conceived idea of the best way forward so that this view is strengthened in debates with colleagues.

Interestingly, our response to debates about empowerment often depends on our definition of 'power' (see also Chapter Five for further discussion). For some people, power is finite – if I have power and give some of it to someone else, then they increase their power and I am less powerful (a 'zero sum game' in which they have 'won' and I have 'lost'). Alternatively, some people see power as infinite – if I share it with someone else, then we are both powerful (a 'win-win' situation). These might be views that we hold subconsciously, without ever having articulated any of this to ourselves. However, people working in health and social care, on reading this section, could try a series of small experiments at work. In situations where you have power compared to someone in need who is trying to access you service, what would happen if you made a conscious decision to share some of your power with others – does this reduce your power, or does everyone benefit?

For present purposes, there are two further issues to consider here:

1. *Individual v collective forms of involvement:* many forms of involvement and empowerment are essentially individual in nature – a worker or a service gathers our individual experiences and/or gives us a say over our own treatment. However, an alternative approach is to think about scope for collective action – bringing people

together to think about services more generally (not just their own treatment) and to work on these issues with others. This can greatly increase the power of potentially marginalised groups – giving people a collective voice, ensuring that people have access to peer support and helping people reflect and learn by comparing their experiences to those of others. Many would argue that some of the most radical changes in health and social care have come about not because of individual patients or their families feeding back on their treatment, but through groups of people coming together to develop a more collective approach.

2. *Consulting versus campaigning*: it is now common for health and social services to seek to 'consult' or 'involve' people in decisions about services – but these can be fairly limited ways of working; positive for some but not sufficient to genuinely change the nature of services or to tackle wider issues. In contrast, another approach is for groups of people using services to adopt a more campaigning approach – not just feeding back to welfare services, but seeking to campaign for specific and positive changes within services (and possibly within wider society too). Thus, individuals from a minority ethnic community who feel that their religious and cultural needs have not been adequately met could feed this back on an individual basis to the people providing their care. However, they could also get together to compare their experiences and feed this back as a group (which might be more likely to influence change than individual feedback alone). Alternatively, they could start to campaign for changes – either with their service providers and/or by drawing attention to the experience of people from minority ethnic communities more generally and by demanding broader social change. A particularly crucial example of this is discussed in Chapter Two, where changes in services for disabled people have been heavily influenced by the campaigning of the **independent living movement** (organisations of disabled people developing alternative ideas about how services should be organised, and campaigning to bring this about). Similar debates have also taken place in mental health services, where further progress might need us to adopt more radical approaches which

seek to challenge social attitudes, stigma and exclusion, rather than just improve a particular service. It is also said that this may be one reason why some services for older people still feel very unmodernised and unambitious compared to some services for other user groups – for various reasons, older people seem to have been slower to form their own collective movement campaigning for change, and many services still seem very traditional. If we wanted a genuinely new approach to funding long-term care (see Chapter Two), for example, older people could feed back their experience of current approaches (although we've known that these experiences are essentially negative for decades). Alternatively, a really organised and fired up movement of older people articulating the need for radical change and campaigning to bring this about could make a significant difference – not least because of the size of the older population and the sheer number of votes it could muster if these issues came to the fore at an election.

Further resources

The Marmot Review (2010) is a very detailed, hard-hitting analysis of **health inequalities** in England, and is essential reading. Internationally, the WHO (2008) *Commission on Social Determinants of Health* is also a key document.

Key **textbooks on health inequalities, health and public health** include:

• Baggott's *Public Health Policy and Politics* (2011) and *Partnerships for Public Health* (2013)
• Hunter's *Partnership Working in Public Health* (Hunter and Perkins, 2014) and *The Public Health System in England* (Hunter et al, 2010)

Although dated, Jones' (1994) book on *The Social Context of Health and Health Work* provides a detailed but accessible overview.

For **social divisions**, see the edited collection by Payne (2013), covering topics such as class, gender, ethnicity, age, childhood, disability, sexuality, religion, poverty and others.

For **user involvement**, there are really useful (usually free) resources, links and guidance produced by organisations such as:

- Healthwatch (www.healthwatch.co.uk)
- Involve (www.invo.org.uk/resource-centre)
- SCIE (www.scie.org.uk)

Glasby et al (2013) have published a free online policy paper about new approaches to adult social care, advocating more **assets-based approaches**. SCIE has published guides to *Asset-based Places* (2017) and to *Growing Innovative Models of Health, Care and Support for Adults* (2018), which summarise a number of promising, small scale, **assets-based approaches** and look at ways to spread such innovation at scale. The Coalition for Collaborative Care has published *A Concise Handbook* for commissioning community development for health (Chanan and Fisher, 2018).

5

Being a professional

While we end up in different roles for all kinds of reasons, lots of people make a positive choice that they want to dedicate themselves to a career in which they can help people and make a real difference. This could be in literally thousands of different ways from being an NHS chief executive to being a cleaner or a porter; being a doctor, a nurse, a physio, a social worker or a care assistant; being an educator or a researcher; and in countless other roles. According to Health Education England, there are over 350 different careers in the NHS, while some 1.48 million people work in the social care sector (see further resources at the end of this chapter for the HEE/NHS Careers website).

To help those thinking about a career in health and social care, this chapter provides an overview of a number of key topics related to health and social care professions, including:

- The nature of professions
- Values and ethics
- Power
- Culture
- Working with others

Professions

Lots of people working in health and social care are 'professionals' in the lay, everyday sense of the term. Depending on the context, this can often mean someone who does what they do for a living (so not an amateur) or someone who is very skilled. However, being a member of a profession means more than just being expert. According to Harvard Business School (Khurana et al, 2005), an occupation is a 'profession' if it meets the following four criteria:

- A common body of knowledge resting on a well-developed, widely accepted theoretical base;
- A system for certifying that individuals possess such knowledge before being licensed or otherwise allowed to practice;
- A commitment to use specialized knowledge for the public good, and a renunciation of the goal of profit maximization, in return for professional autonomy and monopoly power;
- A code of ethics, with provisions for monitoring individual compliance with the code and a system of sanctions for enforcing it.

A similar definition is provided by Professions Australia (see also **Concepts and Debates 5**):

A profession is a disciplined group of individuals who adhere to ethical standards and who hold themselves out as, and are accepted by the public as possessing special knowledge and skills in a widely recognised body of learning derived from research, education and training at a high level, and who are prepared to apply this knowledge and exercise these skills in the interest of others. It is inherent in the definition of a profession that a code of ethics governs the activities of each profession. Such codes require behaviour and practice beyond the personal moral obligations of an individual. They define and demand high standards of behaviour in respect to the services provided to the public and in dealing with professional colleagues. Further, these codes are enforced by the profession and are acknowledged and accepted by the community. (www.professions.com.au/about-us/what-is-a-professional)

Concepts and Debates 5: What is a profession?

The word 'profession' means different things to different people. But at its core, it's meant to be an indicator of trust and expertise.

Traditionally, a 'professional' was someone who derived their income from their expertise or specific talents, as opposed to a hobbyist or amateur. This still carries through to fields today, such as sport.

But given today's fast-changing environment of knowledge and expertise, it's now generally understood that simply deriving an income from a particular task might make you an 'expert' or 'good at your job' – but if you're a 'professional', this has a broader meaning.

There's a long history of attempts to clarify this meaning, and to define the functions of professions. These attempts typically centralise around some sort of moral or ethical foundation within the practice of a specific and usually established expertise ...

Key definitions

*A **profession** is a disciplined group of individuals who adhere to ethical standards. This group positions itself as possessing special knowledge and skills in a widely recognised body of learning derived from research, education and training at a high level, and is recognised by the public as such. A profession is also prepared to apply this knowledge and exercise these skills in the interest of others.*

*A **professional** is a member of a profession. Professionals are governed by codes of ethics, and profess commitment to competence, integrity and morality, altruism, and the promotion of the public good within their expert domain. Professionals are accountable to those served and to society.*

Professionalism comprises the personally held beliefs about one's own conduct as a professional. It's often linked to the upholding of the principles, laws, ethics and conventions of a profession as a way of practice.

Professionalisation is the pattern of how a profession develops, as well as the process of becoming a profession.

Source: Professional Standards Councils, Australia, www.psc.gov.au/what-is-a-profession

In health and social care, there are a number of professions, each of which has its own history, professional body, professional qualifications, codes of conduct and standards. Many also involve a 'protected title' and formal register, so that someone can only call themselves a 'social worker' (for example) if they are professionally qualified and on the register (see **Key Sources 6** for examples from the Health and Care Professions Council). This is important because it means that, when we see a health or social care professional, we feel able to trust them and listen to their advice, safe in the knowledge that they are an expert in their field, that they have appropriate qualifications to do the job and that their competence has been guaranteed by the relevant professional association. The structure of our regulatory bodies is also significant, and social work in England has moved from having its own body (the General Social Care Council) to being one of a number of professions regulated by the Health and Care Professions Council to having a new social work regulator (Social Work England) in a relatively short space of time – with the profession perhaps feeling that these changes indicate a lack of stability and a lack of understanding as to how best recognise the distinctive contribution of social work.

Key Sources 6: Protected titles (Health and Care Professions Council)

The designated titles below are protected by law. Anyone who uses one of these titles must be on our Register. A person who is not registered and who misuses a designated title is breaking the law and may be prosecuted:

Profession	Protected title(s)
Arts therapist	• Art psychotherapist • Art therapist • Dramatherapist • Music therapist
Biomedical scientist	• Biomedical scientist
Chiropodist / podiatrist	• Chiropodist • Podiatrist
Clinical scientist	• Clinical scientist
Dietitian	• Dietitian/Dietician
Hearing aid dispenser	• Hearing aid dispenser
Occupational therapist	• Occupational therapist
Operating department practitioner	• Operating department practitioner
Orthoptist	• Orthoptist
Paramedic	• Paramedic
Physiotherapist	• Physiotherapist • Physical therapist
Practitioner psychologist	• Practitioner psychologist • Registered psychologist • Clinical psychologist • Counselling psychologist • Educational psychologist • Forensic psychologist • Health psychologist • Occupational psychologist • Sport and exercise psychologist
Prosthetist/orthotist	• Prosthetist • Orthotist • Prosthetist and Orthotist
Radiographer	• Radiographer • Diagnostic radiographer • Therapeutic radiographer
Social workers in England	• Social worker
Speech and language therapist	• Speech and language therapist • Speech therapist

Source: Protected titles, HCPC, www.hcpc-uk.org/aboutregistration/protectedtitles

While these definitions seem clear-cut and helpful, there are a number of unresolved tensions in a health and social care context. For example:

1. *Professional vested interests:* health and social care are dominated by a series of different, sometimes very powerful, professions. While this can be a key strength in terms of the training, knowledge and expertise that these groups bring, there can also be tensions between managers and clinicians about the best way of organising services, and it can often be very difficult to bring about change if it is being actively resisted by some of the frontline professions. A good example here is Aneurin Bevan's quote around having to stuff doctors' mouths 'with gold' in order to create the NHS (see Chapter One). It can also be difficult to introduce new, more flexible roles (such as nurse practitioners or physician associates) as these fall outside or blur traditional professional boundaries. To patients, it can sometimes feel as if some services operate according to the convenience of/partly in the interests of the staff who work there, rather than the needs or convenience of people using services (see Chapter Six for further discussion of the relationship between professionals, managers and patients).

2. *The role of nurses:* there are longstanding debates about the nature of the nursing profession, with some claiming that current graduate entry nurses are too far removed from the realities of care-giving (pejoratively described as 'too posh to wash'). While there are significant debates about how best to support staff to deliver compassionate care (see Chapter Six), this feels a really insulting way of framing the debate – implying that some nurses are somehow 'over-educated' for their role and that there is a clear-cut distinction between compassion and intellect. This seems an utterly stupid argument (and it's interesting that this debate has focused on a primarily female workforce, rather than on a male-dominated profession). Given the complexities involved in delivering health and social care in the 21st century, surely we want nurses (and other groups within the workforce) who are clever and caring, capable of analytical and critical thinking, while

at the same time able to carry out practical tasks with skill and compassion? Potentially just as significant is a broader debate about the *nature* of professionalism in nursing. Having long fought for greater recognition of their professional status, nurses have often seemed to make the most progress when they have been taking on aspects of the role of doctors, effectively modelling themselves on a medical notion of what constitutes a good professional. While these are important skills to develop, it would seem a shame if the main way to gain greater professional recognition was to have to be seen to copy medical approaches, rather than having the autonomy to articulate one's own professional contribution and value base.

3. *The nature of management expertise:* there have been longstanding debates as to whether management constitutes a profession. While the topic of management and leadership is discussed in greater detail in Chapter Six, the answer to this question has to be 'no'. Returning to the four criteria outlined above by Harvard Business School, health and social care managers struggle to meet a number of these prerequisites. Rather than a common body of knowledge, managers draw on a range of different knowledge bases, often in a fairly eclectic way. There is no system for certifying that individuals possess such knowledge before they are licensed to practise, and no broadly accepted code of ethics to which managers must subscribe. However, this may be beginning to change, with organisations such as the NHS Leadership Academy seeing their mission as 'professionalising leadership: raising the profile, performance and impact of health system leaders, requiring and supporting them to demonstrate their fit and proper readiness to carry out their leadership role and defining what we expect from them' (www.leadershipacademy.nhs.uk/about/). To do this, the Academy has put in place a series of leadership development programmes for leaders at different levels of seniority and different stages of their career, arguing that health service leaders (whether managers or clinicians by background) should be expected to demonstrate their 'fitness to practise' in just the same way that a doctor or nurse must do. Over time, it is hoped that more and

more leaders will have undertaken such training, creating a new generation of NHS leaders with the skills, behaviours and values needed to respond to current challenges, lead across organisational boundaries and help create the conditions in which staff can be supported to deliver high quality, compassionate care to patients and their families (see **Key Sources 7**).

4. *Professional v organisational regulation*: while individual health and social care professionals are bound by their own professional codes of conduct (discussed further later in the chapter), they also work in organisations that are subject to inspection by national regulators such as (in England) the CQC. These bodies exist to ensure that care is safe and to root out poor practice, but getting the balance right between identifying shortcomings and supporting improvement can be difficult, and the process of being inspected can sometimes feel very stressful and overwhelming (see **Voices of Experience 8** for an example). Health and social care professions are therefore subject to multiple forms of regulation and can have their practice scrutinised by a range of different bodies. While each of these mechanisms is designed to achieve positive outcomes for people using services, multiple and overlapping forms of accountability, inspection and regulation can also create significant pressures.

Key Sources 7: Professionalising leadership in the NHS

The [NHS Leadership] Academy approach follows a well-established model in industry where talent is identified, managed and developed to create an effective succession pipeline for key roles.

In the NHS we have increasing challenges identifying senior leaders able and ready to take on some of the more enduringly complex roles in challenged NHS organisations. Much work is being done to create a temporary solution to this shortage, but the problem is one of sustained underinvestment in developing skilled leaders at every level in the NHS. Without a more structured, robust and informed strategy to address this problem we will need to keep undertaking short term fixes to find the right candidates for key roles.

The Academy is in a position where the complexity of a leadership role is more understood, and we are working with two internationally respected consortia able to deliver high quality leadership training and skills development, in the context of healthcare. Having the right number and quality of leaders at every level is no accident and the NHS needs to be at least as rigorous in developing talent as any other industry. Our programmes ensure people are properly trained to fulfil the roles they aspire to and there is more likelihood of a more consistent level of success in these roles. It also creates a more robust pipeline of talent, who have properly gained skills, experience and competence in their roles, have a structured and assessed development programme matched to their career progression and so a greater degree of confidence in securing a more senior role.

The professional leadership programmes form the Academy's main intervention to achieve the professionalisation of leadership in healthcare – to insist that leaders are properly developed to qualify them for leadership roles before taking them up. If leaders are ever to be taken seriously in their roles, if the profession is to be recognised as a crucial contributor to a great health service rather than a burdensome cost then the discharging of leaders' roles and responsibilities should carry the same requirements for demonstration of fitness to practice, as other professions across the NHS.

Source: NHS Leadership Academy, Professionalisation of leadership, www.leadershipacademy.nhs.uk/blog/professionalisation-leadership

Although much less well-resourced than in the NHS, there are also a series of social care leaders programmes – see www.skillsforcare.org.uk/Leadership-management/Leadership-programmes/Leadership-programmes.aspx

Voices of Experience 8: Being inspected

In 2017, the GP magazine, *Pulse*, set out two differing experiences of the inspection process. These are the perceptions of two different GPs (one positive and one negative), and we don't know what the inspectors would say about the same visits. However, the two quotes below illustrate some of the highs and lows of being inspected, and the impact it can have on individual staff.

Was your CQC inspection a good experience?

"Yes – it was good on the whole, although we started off somewhat fearful. We came in at a weekend and went through everything to ensure compliance. On the day, I talked at the poor inspector incessantly for hours – he looked exhausted. The pharmacy inspector was so impressed with what our pharmacist had done, he left early. We employed a locum to see patients for the day to free us up. A stream of patients came in, all with positive things to say. We received a 'good' rating. We treated the inspectors with kindness and courtesy, were open to their feedback, and had everything they needed to hand well in advance. It gave us a good reason to spring clean and introduce a lot of positive changes. Our staff got a morale boost."

"No – we prepared for the inspection and were confident our presentation would go down well but we were faced with inspectors who just did not understand what they were dealing with. We listed all our unique achievements, like an eating disorder service, a day bed unit for students and a highly successful meningitis campaign. Despite this the inspectors implied we would only get a rating of 'requires improvement' partly because we hadn't mentioned alcohol – which we do treat as part of routine care. I was speechless. It was the worst day of my career. I had to come in on my day off and spend eight hours typing out an 11-page document challenging them. In the end, the only criticism they had

> was that we didn't have photocopies of all the locums' IDs – but patients aren't put in danger because we don't have a photocopy of a document. The inspections are completely bureaucratic. I received an apology letter in the end. The inspection was in March, it wasn't sorted until early August; I didn't sleep properly for three months after it. It cost hours and hours of time that I could have spent on patient care."
>
> Source: *Pulse*, 5 May 2017: www.pulsetoday.co.uk/your-practice/regulation/was-your-cqc-inspection-a-good-experience/20034393.article

Values and ethics

Part of being a professional is to practise according to a set of values or ethics – moral principles which govern our behaviour and decisions. Within the NHS, a key document is the **NHS Constitution**, which sets out the rights of patients, the public and staff, together with a series of underpinning values and a set of standards which health services try to meet (see **Key Sources 8**). Unfortunately, there is no comparable document for adult social care, although a definition of social work from the International Federation of Social Workers emphasises a number of key principles that underpin the profession:

Social work is a practice-based profession and an academic discipline that promotes social change and development, social cohesion, and the empowerment and liberation of people. Principles of social justice, human rights, collective responsibility and respect for diversities are central to social work. Underpinned by theories of social work, social sciences, humanities and indigenous knowledges, social work engages people and structures to address life challenges and enhance wellbeing. (www.ifsw.org/what-is-social-work/global-definition-of-social-work/)

Key Sources 8: The NHS Constitution

Seven key principles guide the NHS in all it does. They are underpinned by core NHS values which have been derived from extensive discussions with staff, patients and the public ...:

- *The NHS provides a comprehensive service, available to all*
- *Access to NHS services is based on clinical need, not an individual's ability to pay*
- *The NHS aspires to the highest standards of excellence and professionalism*
- *The patient will be at the heart of everything the NHS does*
- *The NHS works across organisational boundaries*
- *The NHS is committed to providing best value for taxpayers' money*
- *The NHS is accountable to the public, communities and patients that it serves*

NHS values:

Working together for patients – *patients come first in everything we do. We fully involve patients, staff, families, carers, communities, and professionals inside and outside the NHS. We put the needs of patients and communities before organisational boundaries. We speak up when things go wrong.*

Respect and dignity – *we value every person – whether patient, their families or carers, or staff – as an individual, respect their aspirations and commitments in life, and seek to understand their priorities, needs, abilities and limits. We take what others have to say seriously. We are honest and open about our point of view and what we can and cannot do.*

Commitment to quality of care – *we earn the trust placed in us by insisting on quality and striving to get the basics of quality of care – safety, effectiveness and patient experience – right every time. We encourage and welcome feedback from patients, families, carers,* staff and the public. We use this to improve the care we provide and build on our successes.

Compassion – we ensure that compassion is central to the care we provide and respond with humanity and kindness to each person's pain, distress, anxiety or need. We search for the things we can do, however small, to give comfort and relieve suffering. We find time for patients, their families and carers, as well as those we work alongside. We do not wait to be asked, because we care.

Improving lives – we strive to improve health and wellbeing and people's experiences of the NHS. We cherish excellence and professionalism wherever we find it – in the everyday things that make people's lives better as much as in clinical practice, service improvements and innovation. We recognise that all have a part to play in making ourselves, patients and our communities healthier.

Everyone counts – we maximise our resources for the benefit of the whole community, and make sure nobody is excluded, discriminated against or left behind. We accept that some people need more help, that difficult decisions have to be taken – and that when we waste resources we waste opportunities for others.

Source: The NHS Constitution for England, www.gov.uk/government/publications/the-nhs-constitution-for-england/the-nhs-constitution-for-england

Beyond these more general statements, individual professional bodies and regulators often set out more detailed codes of conduct or lists of professional values. Thus, the General Medical Council (2014) publishes the standards expected of every doctor on the register, the British Association of Social Workers has a *Code of Ethics for Social Work* (2014) and the Nursing and Midwifery Council has a code of *Professional Standards of Practice and Behaviour* (2015). The British Medical Association also publishes guidance on ethics via a number of handbooks and an online 'A to Z' (from abortion, access to health records and advance decision making to victims of forced marriage, vulnerable adults and withholding and withdrawing life-prolonging medical treatment; www.bma.org.uk/advice/employment/ethics/ethics-a-to-z).

Typically, the different health and social care professions have guidance and standards provided by two different types of body:

1. The *statutory regulator*, which seeks to protect the public, register members of the profession and maintain standards (such as the General Medical Council, the Nursing and Midwifery Council and the Health and Care Professions Council) – a body external to the profession to guarantee standards.
2. The profession's own trade union/professional body (such as the British Medical Association, the Royal College of Nursing, the British Association of Social Workers, and others) – a form of *self-regulation*, with the profession itself taking a lead in promoting good conduct and upholding its own standards.

If a health or social care professional falls short of these codes/standards, they can be referred to the regulator and can face a series of different sanctions – including being forbidden from practising any more and being taken off the register.

While each of these professional codes is slightly different, they tend to cover similar ground. For example, a common framework in medical ethics is set out by US philosophers Beauchamp and Childress (2012) in their textbook on *Principles of Biomedical Ethics* (see **Voices of Experience 9**). This outlines four key moral principles:

- Respect for autonomy (patients have the right to make choices about their treatment, including the right to refuse treatment)
- Beneficence (acting in the best interests of the patient)
- Non-maleficence (doing no harm)
- Justice (fairness and equality)

Voices of Experience 9: Ethics in practice

The UK Clinical Ethics Network sets out a case study to illustrate the four principles of biomedical ethics in practice:

Mrs Y is 56 years old and has a learning disability. She is admitted to hospital with an ovarian cyst. The cyst is blocking her ureter and if left untreated will result in renal failure. Mrs Y would need an operation to remove the cyst. Mrs Y has indicated quite clearly that she does not want a needle inserted for the anaesthetic for the operation to remove the cyst – she is uncomfortable in a hospital setting and is frightened of needles.

The clinician is concerned that if the cyst is not removed Mrs Y will develop renal failure and require dialysis which would involve the regular use of needles and be very difficult to carry out given her fear of needles and discomfort with hospitals. The anaesthetist is concerned that if Mrs Y does not comply with the procedure then she would need to be physically restrained. Mrs Y's niece visits her in the care home every other month. The niece is adamant that her aunt should receive treatment. Should the surgeon perform the operation despite Mrs Y's objections?

Respect for autonomy: *the principle of respect for autonomy entails taking into account and giving consideration to the patient's views on his/her treatment. Autonomy is not an all or nothing concept. Mrs Y may not be fully autonomous (and not legally competent to refuse treatment) but this does not mean that ethically her views should not be considered and respected as far as possible. She has expressed her wishes clearly; she does not want a needle inserted for the anaesthetic. An autonomous decision does not have to be the 'correct' decision from an objective viewpoint otherwise individual needs and values would not be respected. However an autonomous decision is one that is informed – has Mrs Y been given enough information, in a manner that she can comprehend?*

Beneficence: *the healthcare professional should act to benefit his/her patient. This principle may clash with the principle of respect for autonomy when the patient makes a decision that the healthcare professional does not think will benefit the patient – is not in her best interests. Here we should consider both the long-term and short-term effects of overriding Mrs Y's views. In the short-term Mrs Y will be frightened to have a needle inserted in her arm and to be in hospital – this may lead her to distrust healthcare professionals in the future and to be reluctant to seek medical help. In the long-term there will be a benefit to Mrs Y in having her autonomy overridden on this occasion. Without treatment she will suffer serious and long-term health problems that would require greater medical intervention (ongoing dialysis) than the treatment required now (operation). The benefits of acting beneficently would need to be weighed against the dis-benefits of failing to respect Mrs Y's autonomy. (From a legal point of view the wishes of a competent patient cannot be overridden in his best interests).*

Non-maleficence: *do no harm to the patient. Here, Mrs Y would be harmed by forcibly restraining her in order to insert the needle for anaesthesia. On the other hand if she is not treated now she will require ongoing dialysis a number of times per week. If she does not comply with dialysis it would be impractical to administer and may require restraint. Which course of action would result in the greatest harm? This assessment relies on assumptions: how successful is the operation likely to be; how likely will Mrs Y comply with dialysis?*

Justice: *it would be relevant to consider cost effectiveness of the treatment options for Mrs Y, and the impact the decision about her treatment has on the availability of treatment for others (awaiting dialysis).*

Source: Ethical Frameworks, UKCEN, www.ukcen.net/ethical_issues/ ethical_frameworks/the_four_principles_of_biomedical_ethics

The general principles set out above are often supplemented by additional principles concerning respect for the individual/treating people with dignity and honesty (including in situations where something has gone wrong). As an example, the Nursing and Midwifery Council and the General Medical Council have published a joint statement of professional values (see **Key Sources 9**).

Key Sources 9: Nursing and Midwifery Council and General Medical Council – Joint statement of professional values

Nurses and doctors share professional values. These are set out in the NMC's code: 'Standards of conduct, performance and ethics for nurses and midwives' and in the GMC's 'Duties of a doctor'.

Nurses, midwives and doctors agree to:

- *Make the care of people [patients, clients, service users] their first concern*
- *Treat people as individuals and respect their dignity*
- *Act without delay if they believe that they, or a colleague, or the environment in which they are providing care, is putting someone at risk ...*

Doctors, nurses and midwives are expected to:

- *Be kind and considerate to those for whom they provide care, and to their carers and families*
- *Listen to, and work in partnership with those for whom they provide care*
- *Work constructively with colleagues to provide patient-centred care, recognising that multidisciplinary teamwork, encouraging constructive challenge from all team members, safety-focused leadership and a culture based on openness and learning when things go wrong are fundamental to achieve high quality care*
- *Follow their employing or contracting bodies' procedures when they have concerns about the safety or dignity of people receiving care*

> • *Be open and honest with people receiving care if something goes wrong.*
>
> *The challenges facing doctors, nurses and midwives today are very different from those faced by their predecessors but the human values which underpin these professions remain constant and those values underpin the trust which lies at the heart of the doctor–patient, nurse–patient relationship.*
>
> Source: Nursing and Midwifery Council and General Medical Council (2012)

Power

In Chapter Four, there was a discussion of the nature of power and developments in terms of **user involvement** and **empowerment**. Being a professional often means being in a position of power – and having a code of conduct or a set of professional and ethical values (see above) influences how we choose to exercise this power. While health and social services often care for people in need, there are a number of situations when they can exert significant control over people's lives. For example, if a person with a mental health problem is assessed as being a risk to themselves or to others, they can be 'sectioned' (admitted to hospital, potentially against their will, for assessment and/or treatment). In children's services, social workers can seek a court order for a child to be taken away from their parents and placed 'in care'. For these reasons, various care professions (but perhaps particularly social work) embrace both 'care' and 'control', and can be viewed ambiguously by members of the public. While we like 'care', we sometimes feel less positively about 'control' (especially if it us that's being controlled).

At the same time, some members of the public may feel that social workers (or other health and social care professionals) are not doing enough to control the behaviour of some people. A good example of this might be in the case of a child death or a mental health homicide, where there can be searching questions about whether health and social services should have intervened differently or earlier. This can cause significant complexities, not least in light of the principle of autonomy (and the right to refuse treatment) set out above. Certainly, when I was training as a social worker, I encountered a number of situations where a frail older person was struggling to care for themselves at home. Whereas the family or a doctor might want the person to go into a care home, the older person often wanted to remain at home, and this was their choice. I certainly didn't have the power to 'force' the person to go into a home against their wishes (even if I'd wanted to), and my role was more about making sure that the person understood the options available to them (and the consequences of these) and that they were as well supported as possible, irrespective of the decision they made. This tended not to go down well with the person's family or their doctor, who assumed that I had more power than was actually the case, and that I could 'make' the older person do something they didn't want to do.

Alongside very formal, statutory powers, health and social care professionals have all kinds of day-to-day, administrative and informal powers, including:

- deciding who might be eligible for treatment or for a service;
- deciding whether something is urgent or can afford to wait;
- deciding whether to involve other people in the case or to refer elsewhere.

Moreover, professionals are often trusted by their patients and service users, who often depend on the individual practitioner whom they encounter to provide meaningful information about the options available. Thus, the advice and information we give, the range of options we provide and the way in which we articulate what may be possible can have a significant impact on what the person then does. For example, in setting out someone's options, I might say: 'You can choose between X and Y. (There's also option Z, but I don't think that would work very well for you) – which of X or Y do you want to choose?' In this scenario, it is highly unlikely that many people would choose option Z, so the way I frame the options has effectively narrowed the person's choice from the very beginning.

This is a very powerful and responsible position to be in – and it's an incredible privilege that individuals and broader society place so much trust in health and social care professionals. This makes it crucial that we use our power well – hence the importance of the professional ethics and values set out above.

Culture

Different health and social care practitioners undertake different functions and have different skills – but they also have different organisational and professional cultures. Culture is often defined as 'the way we do things round here' (Ouchi and Johnson, 1978) – and can be a shorthand term for how a group of people see themselves and the world around them, how they dress, how they speak, how they behave, and so on. Without suggesting that we're all the same just because we do the same job, most readers could walk into a room full of doctors, nurses, social workers or managers and make a fairly accurate guess as to which group they had joined within a few seconds of talking to people. Like the earlier discussion around the assumptions we make and the stereotypes we hold about others (see Chapter Four), this can be helpful if it's a shorthand for understanding the world around us, but can also be extremely unhelpful if we make such assumptions uncritically.

As an example, Carpenter (1995) explores the perceptions which medical and nursing students hold of each other, and the extent to which these can be challenged by interprofessional education. Medical students saw nurses as caring, dedicated, moderately good communicators and 'do gooders', while nursing students saw doctors as dedicated, confident and decisive – but also as arrogant, detached and poor communicators. Having spent time with each other in interprofessional education settings, some of the more negative of these views had started to change. Similarly, **Voices of Experience 10** sets out some of the perceptions which health and social care staff from mental health backgrounds have of each other (Peck and Crawford, 2002, 2004). While many people working in health and social care would query whether these observations are 'true', the fact that colleagues perceived them to be true says something about how we see ourselves and others, how we respond to people from different backgrounds to our own and how we find ways to collaborate across professional boundaries when people have complex, cross-cutting needs.

Voices of Experience 10: Professional and organisational culture

Peck and Crawford (2002, 2004) asked staff from health and social services what they admired about each other and what they did not understand about the other agency/profession. Extracts from this work included (2004, p 10):

Saying 'no' – *Health staff perceived social services as being able to say 'no' to individuals through the use of eligibility criteria whereas, because the NHS is 'universal' and 'free at the point of delivery', they are unable to say 'no'. Social services personnel perceived themselves as being unable to say 'no' to society, whereas the NHS was seen as being there to deal with specific and defined problems ...*

Training and supervision – *NHS staff assumed that social services have effective and well-resourced practitioner supervision whereas health did not. Social services staff thought that health meant the same by the term 'supervision' as they did, and were surprised that supervision did not appear to be as rigorous. This was just one example of health and social services being represented as two organisations separated by a common language ...*

Power relationships – *health colleagues found it difficult to understand the nuances of political decision-making and the benefits of well-established relationships between elected members and officers. Social services staff did not understand the relationship between doctors and managers in the NHS, finding the inability of managers to make doctors adopt standard procedures inexplicable and frustrating.*

Decision-making processes – *social services staff saw local government as striving to be inclusive and consultative. They saw this as a democratic strength. Health staff, in contrast, saw it as a source of delay. Decision-making in the NHS was mutually recognised as being less formal and usually quicker.*

Working with others

Following on from the discussion of culture above, a core part of being a health or social care profession is about working with others – either in teams within our own organisation and/or across organisational boundaries. A leading researcher and commentator with regards to teamworking is Michael West (2012). While lots of roles in health and social care require people to work on their own initiative, to take responsibility for their own practice and, in some roles, to be out and about in the community as lone workers, the vast majority of our time in health and social care organisations is spent in teams. Moreover, the quality of our experience in such teams can vary significantly, from 'real teams' (where people feel they are part of the team, agree on team objectives and work closely and interdependently with other team members) to 'pseudo teams' (where people don't agree on their shared objectives, aren't sure who is/isn't a member of the team, and who work separately or towards different goals). All the available evidence suggests that working in supportive and successful teams is crucial to individual and collective well-being, the quality of care we deliver and the extent to which we are able to learn and innovate. Although our person specifications usually focus primarily on individual knowledge, skills and experience, we are all interdependent on others and we forget this at our peril. As West explains:

I think the most important finding or understanding that we have from our 30 year programme of research is that the team is the basic unit of production for human beings – this is the way that we've always worked, lived, loved and raised our young – in teams and small groups. And this form of working has enabled us to achieve remarkable things – to uncover the structure of the human genome and to explore the beginnings of the universe. Our challenge is to recreate that form of working effectively in modern, large organisations.

First of all we need to be clear about which tasks need teams. Then it's really important that every team has a limited number of clear, shared, challenging objectives, that everybody is clear about their role and each other's role in the team, that they work interdependently as a team – closely together, and that they meet regularly to review their performance and how they can improve their performance. When we have these basics in place, we can go on to develop decision making, communication, constructive debate and inter-team working.

When we compare organisations that have really well developed team work with organisations that have poor team work what we see is that in the case of the latter organisations, there are many more errors, there's much less learning, there are lower levels of innovation. Moreover staff stress is higher, roles are much less clear and people don't feel the social support that they get from working in effective teams. So there are really big differences in terms of productivity, innovation, staff well-being and staff engagement between organisations that have good team working and those that have poor or no team working. (Why Teams? AOD, www.astonod.com/library)

While some teams may be made up of people from the same role or professional background, lots of health and social care involves working with people from different organisational or professional backgrounds. This is discussed in greater detail in Chapter Three, but **Key Sources 10** provides an example of just some of the ways in which Health Education England (the national body responsible for education and training in health care) describes the changing nature of what it means to be a professional in an era of interagency working. In the past, many of us were trained to work in individual professions, spending the bulk of our time with students and practitioners from our own professional background, and seeking to learn from and emulate the practice of people in similar roles to our own. This is important for inducting oneself into a chosen profession, but (by itself) it can also be a very limited way to understand the world. Whatever the future holds, today's professionals and those of tomorrow are going to have to work across agency and professional boundaries to an even greater extent than in the past, and the ability to do this successfully is likely to be highly prized.

Key Sources 10: Working together in new ways/roles

According to Health Education England:

Many staff now work in roles that cover both health and social care, and the values and qualities needed are very similar.

The Government has set out the need for the health and social care sectors to develop new integrated care models to promote health and wellbeing and provide care. In the future, this could mean your career crossing both sectors in new and exciting roles.

Several methods are in place across the country to develop and promote these new ways of working, such as:

- *providing key skills training for health staff so they can assess mental health wellbeing*
- *training for physiotherapists so they can undertake dementia assessments*
- *enhancing the competencies of care home staff so they can support clinical and non-clinical professionals*
- *ways of encouraging closer working and learning between primary and community-based nursing teams.*

Source: Working in social care, NHS Health Education England, www. healthcareers.nhs.uk/working-health/working-social-care

Further resources

Health Education England has a website on **working in the NHS** (including sections on 'health systems across the UK' and 'working in social care'), with material on how the NHS is structured, what kinds of people it needs, careers, pay and benefits (see www.healthcareers. nhs.uk/working-health).

In England, national bodies such as **Skills for Care** (www. skillsforcare.org.uk) and **Skills for Health** (www.skillsforhealth.org. uk) are the sector skills councils for health and social care, seeking to develop a sustainable workforce for the care sector.

In health care, the **NHS Constitution** is a key document, setting out the rights that patients, the public and staff are entitled to, and the pledges that the NHS is committed to achieving (www.gov. uk/government/publications/the-nhs-constitution-for-england/ the-nhs-constitution-for-england).

In England, key **professional regulators** include:

• The General Medical Council (www.gmc-uk.org)
• The Health and Care Professions Council (www.hcpc-uk.co.uk)
• The Nursing and Midwifery Council (www.nmc.org.uk)

A guide to **working across agency boundaries** is published by Policy Press as part of their 'Better Partnership Working' series (Glasby and Dickinson, 2014). There are also books on *Interprofessional Education and Training* (Carpenter and Dickinson, 2016) and *Working in Teams* (Jelphs et al, 2016) as part of this series.

Peck and Crawford's (2002) article on **cultural differences between health and social care** is a helpful illustration of the impact of professional differences and stereotypes, while their 2004 guide to *'Culture' in Partnerships* is a helpful overview of what we mean by the concept of 'culture' and what we can do about it.

Michael West (2012) is a leading expert on **teamworking**, and lots of his articles, reports, blogs, presentations and videos are available to access free online, including via the AOD website (www.affinoad. com/library/) and the King's Fund (www.kingsfund.org.uk/about-us/ whos-who/michael-west).

6

Delivering care

Preceding chapters have looked at how health and social care are organised, how they are funded, their history and some of their key features. These are important issues, as these factors continue to shape current services and what might be possible next. Understanding the broader context also helps people using services, working in care settings or even as voters and taxpayers to understand the bigger picture, and to play an active part in ongoing debates about how we can improve the care we deliver.

At the same time, people working in health and social care still have ill or frail people coming through the front door and have no choice but to keep on delivering care as best they can, almost irrespective of some of the issues discussed above. If you're a busy nurse in an A&E department as the victim of a serious car accident is wheeled in, the priority is saving the person's life and giving them the best chance of recovering – however one's service is funded or organised or relates to other agencies. With this in mind, this chapter looks at the realities of delivering care, including discussion of:

- Management and leadership
- The different perspectives of patients/service users, welfare professionals and managers
- New models of care
- Job satisfaction, stress and care as emotional labour
- Skills and training
- The future workforce and seven day services

Management and leadership

While clinicians (especially doctors) have long played a significant role in the design and management of health services, an official review by the then Conservative government led to the growth of **general management** within the NHS from the early 1980s onwards (see **Key Sources 11**). Since then, there has been a significant increase in the number of managers and senior leaders, not least as budgets have continued to expand, as needs have risen and as complexity has increased.

Key Sources 11: General management in the NHS

We were brought in not to be instant experts on all aspects of the NHS but, because of our business experience, to advise on the management of the NHS. We have been told that the NHS is different from business in management terms, not least because the NHS is not concerned with the profit motive and must be judged by wider social standards which cannot be measured. These differences can be greatly overstated. The clear similarities between NHS management and business management are much more important. In many organisations in the private sector, profit does not immediately impinge on large numbers of managers below Board level. They are concerned with levels of service, quality of product, meeting budgets, cost improvement, productivity, motivating and rewarding staff, research and development, and the long term viability of the undertaking. All things that parliament is urging on the NHS. In the private sector the results in all these areas would normally be carefully monitored against pre-determined standards and objectives.

The NHS does not have the profit motive, but it is, of course, enormously concerned with control of expenditure. Surprisingly, however, it still lacks any real continuous evaluation of its performance against criteria such as those set out above. Rarely are precise management objectives set; there is little measurement of health output; clinical evaluation of particular practices is by no means common and economic evaluation of those practices extremely rare. Nor can the NHS display a ready assessment of the effectiveness with which it is meeting the needs and expectations of the people it serves. Businessmen have a keen sense of how well they are looking after their customers. Whether the NHS is meeting the needs of the patient, and the community, and can prove that it is doing so, is open to question ...

One of our most immediate observations from a business background is the lack of a clearly defined general management function throughout the NHS. By general management we mean the responsibility drawn together in one person, at different levels of the organisation, for planning, implementation and control of performance. The NHS is one of the largest undertakings in Western Europe. It requires enormous resources; its role is very politically sensitive; it demands top class management ...

At no level is the general management role clearly being performed by an identifiable individual. In short if Florence Nightingale were carrying her lamp through the corridors of the NHS today she would almost certainly be searching for the people in charge.

Absence of this general management support means that there is no driving force seeking and accepting direct and personal responsibility for developing management plans, securing their implementation and monitoring actual achievement. It means that the process of devolution of responsibility, including discharging responsibility to the Units [units of management or areas of service], is far too slow. The centre is still too much involved in too many of the wrong things and too little involved in some that really matter. For example, local management must be allowed to determine its own needs for information, with higher management drawing on that information for its own purposes. The Units and the Authorities are being swamped with directives without being given direction. Lack of the general management responsibility also means that certain major initiatives are difficult to implement.

Source: Griffiths review, 1983, www.nhshistory.net/griffiths.html

Over time, these changes have led to a series of accusations that the NHS has too many managers, with an implication (in the tabloids in particular) that we may be wasting money through too much bureaucracy and by employing too many well-paid people in roles which are sometimes portrayed as largely irrelevant to the delivery of patient care. Leaving aside the fact that some of the highest-paid individuals can be senior clinicians rather than general managers, this is still an insulting and short-sighted debate. Contrary to popular misconceptions, all the available evidence suggests that the NHS is under- rather than over-managed, with a smaller managerial workforce and relatively low management costs when compared to other sectors of the economy and other health systems (see, for example, King's Fund, 2011). This is despite the fact that the NHS is subject to multiple and overlapping systems of regulation, audit, inspection and accreditation – mostly set up by national government to satisfy itself with NHS performance:

> Politicians of all parties who criticise the level of bureaucracy within the NHS should recognise that they cannot have their cake and eat it. Some of the things they desire of the future health service – greater transparency, comparable performance data to inform choice, drive accountability and improve quality – all come at a cost. (King's Fund, 2011, p 2)

Overall, the King's Fund (2011, pp 1–2 and 23) concludes that:

> In most of business, the requirement for good management is almost a given. No company would reckon to stand a chance of running well without it. Publicly quoted companies are assessed by analysts in part on the quality of their leadership and management. Yet in the public sector – and in the NHS in particular – whenever politicians talk about management it is almost invariably a pejorative term. It is often equated sneeringly with bureaucracy. Whole political careers have been built on attacking it. Alan Milburn [then health secretary] ... first made his name as an opposition health spokesman by attacking the

'men in grey suits' who he reckoned had proliferated as a result of the Conservatives' introduction of an internal market in health care. Recently, Anne Milton, [then] health minister, derided primary care staff who are currently responsible for around £80 billion of NHS spend as 'pen pushers' ...

The public is no more sympathetic. Perhaps it takes its cue from the political attacks on bureaucracy. A recent poll conducted by Ipsos MORI ... showed that 85 per cent of the public supported proposals to reduce the number of managers in the NHS by one-third.

Yet the distinction between the 'front line' and management, or between 'front line' and 'back office', is far from helpful. No surgeon will operate efficiently without a theatre manager. No general practitioner can see patients without a receptionist to arrange appointments and a manager to look after budgets, staff and buildings. And no public health department can prepare for emergencies or plan for a flu pandemic without excellent planning.

Consider a 999 call centre: at what point does which part of the service cease to be 'front line'? The call taker clearly is. But they cannot operate without an office to sit in and information and communication technology that enables the despatch of police, fire and ambulance staff. They need well-maintained vehicles if the public is to receive an effective service. Yet most people would not describe information software and vehicle maintenance as front line.

[Overall] leadership and management in the NHS matter, and the role of managers should be celebrated and not undermined.

While similar issues exist in adult social care, it is interesting that most public debate has focused on the NHS (presumably because of its political importance and the amount of public and media scrutiny it receives).

The different perspectives of patients/service users, professionals and managers

Following on from the above debates, the delivery of health and social care has often been significantly influenced by the different perspectives and contributions of patients/service users, frontline professionals and managers. Chapters Two and Four set out the changes that have taken place in the role which people using services want to play in the design and delivery of services, moving from a paternalistic ethos and a passive role, to one in which people expect to have a say over how care is delivered, and can even receive funding with which to design their own support. Similarly, the section above has outlined the growth of management and leadership within previously clinically-led public services, recognising that this is a crucial aspect of delivering excellent care. At its best, this could mean that we have really engaged patients and service users (who are experts by experience and in what works for them) taking a lead in managing their own health and well-being; really well trained and supported health and social care professionals delivering amazing care; and really well-organised and well-led services. However, there is also scope for these different groups to have different interests and different views on how best to deliver care, with corresponding scope for tension, disagreement and jockeying for position. For example, in social care, some social workers have been active champions of the **personalisation agenda** (see Chapter Two), while others have been concerned about a potential loss of social work values and identity. In the NHS, there has been a much slower start around personalisation, with significant concerns about what might happen if patients have greater control over their own care (perhaps reflecting different perspectives on risk, the nature of clinical expertise and the role of people using services). In both health and social care, frontline practitioners have sometimes felt that senior managers do not understand the realities of delivering care and may be too concerned with money and with very narrow notions of performance. Equally, senior leaders may perceive some clinicians as more concerned with their own particular service or individual status than with the needs of the whole population/system. Some of these issues are captured in a fascinating blog and video by the then Chief Executive of the NHS in England, Sir David Nicholson (see **Voices of Experience 11**), reviewing the implications of the 2012 health reforms, the impact of austerity and the changing nature of our relationships over time.

Voices of Experience 11: Patients, professionals and managers

Working in the NHS, the last 40 years have seen many challenges for managers like me. They've spanned a range of issues, but what they all have in common is the interplay between clinicians, managers and patients and the broader economic circumstances of the time.

In the early 1970s, there was a radical Conservative government committed to reforming the NHS. The financial context was also very challenging, with interventions by the International Monetary Fund and the introduction of 'cash limiting.' Up until this point, clinicians could effectively seek funding for whatever they wanted to do, and it was from this moment on that greater financial awareness was needed in order for us to meet rising need within more constrained budgets.

In the 1980s, the first Griffiths review placed general managers rather than clinicians at the heart of the system – although the role of patients remained limited. In one sense it wasn't until 'The NHS Plan' in 2000 that the views of patients – about access and waiting times, for example – became more influential (often through politicians examining the polling data and using this to construct the 'must do' targets of the day). Ironically, this led to even greater power for managers as the implementers of government targets – and patients were still only really represented indirectly via the targets set by national government.

Following the Health and Social Care Act, the financial and political context has parallels with the early 1970s – although arguably the scale of challenge is even greater. After many years of additional investment, the international economic outlook has changed, and we are going to have to get used to doing much more with little or no growth in budgets. This is going to have to involve patients, clinicians and managers working together in new ways.

For me, there are three main pillars that we need to build on:

1. *Clinical commissioning: GPs are at the heart of the health service, and play a crucial role in people's lives and in local communities. The decisions they make also impact on almost all other parts of the system, and it is vital that GPs are at the forefront of the current changes. However, GP by themselves aren't enough – and we need nurses, allied health professionals and all the primary health care team involved in greater clinical commissioning and leadership.*
2. *The financial challenges we face are such that we cannot focus only on our own profession or our own organisation. We will have to find ways of working together more effectively across primary, community and acute care. Clinical senates [independent committees providing expert clinical advice to commissioners] will therefore be an important forum to break down traditional barriers and to develop more joined-up responses to need.*
3. *The role of the public is crucial – and local government (via Health and Wellbeing Boards) has an essential role in terms of providing local leadership, joining up care and prioritising local needs...*

Source: Sir David Nicholson, Chief Executive of the NHS in England, HSMC Health Policy Lecture, 40 years of change in the NHS, www.birmingham.ac.uk/research/perspective/change-NHS-nicholson.aspx

New models of care

A good example of a situation where people using services, professionals and managers all have a role to play is around the new models of care being developed in different parts of the health and social care system. Responding to an ageing population, rising need and a challenging financial context, local and national leaders have increasingly looked to new ways of delivering care in order to meet needs more effectively. In one sense, this has been a consistent theme throughout this book (and the history of health and social care more generally) – and other periods of national or financial crisis have seen dramatic reforms (not least the creation of the NHS itself after the Second World War). In recent years, however, examples of new models of care have included:

- a focus on **micro-enterprise** and **assets-based approaches** to adult social care, set out in Chapter Four;
- ongoing attempts to integrate health and social care (see Chapter Three);
- the creation of NHS **Foundation Trusts** in the early to mid-2000s to give high-performing NHS organisations greater freedom from central control and flexibility;
- the movement of some traditional public services into new ownership structures – for example, via moving some health and social care into **social enterprises** (voluntary organisations which operate on a more commercial basis, using any surpluses they generate to reinvest in their social mission) or employee-led organisations (with staff playing a greater role in the ownership and governance of organisations – perhaps via a cooperative model).

However, at the time of writing, there is significant activity underway in England in response to the vision set out in the *NHS Five Year Forward View* (NHS England, 2014) – see **Key Sources 12**.

Key Sources 12: New models of care

STPs and integrated care systems

In 2016, NHS organisations and local councils came together to form 44 Sustainability and Transformation Partnerships (STPs) covering the whole of England, and set out their proposals to improve health and care for patients. In some areas, a partnership will evolve to form an integrated care system, a new type of even closer collaboration. In an integrated care system, NHS organisations, in partnership with local councils and others, take collective responsibility for managing resources, delivering NHS standards, and improving the health of the population they serve.

Local services can provide better and more joined-up care for patients when different organisations work together in this way. For staff, improved collaboration can help to make it easier to work with colleagues from other organisations. And systems can better understand data about local people's health, allowing them to provide care that is tailored to individual needs. By working alongside councils, and drawing on the expertise of others such as local charities and community groups, the NHS can help people to live healthier lives for longer, and to stay out of hospital when they do not need to be there. In return, integrated care system leaders gain greater freedoms to manage the operational and financial performance of services in their area. They will draw on the experience of the 50 'vanguard' sites, which have led the development of new care models across the country ...

The first wave of integrated care systems are already assuming accountability for local operational and financial performance. From April 2018, they will begin to gain new financial flexibilities and to use new tools for better understanding local health data. Further integrated care systems will be confirmed by NHS England and NHS Improvement in 2018. To become one, a local system must show its partnership is advanced enough to make shared decisions, improve services for the public and manage resources collectively. (NHS England, Integrated care systems, www.england. nhs.uk/accountable-care-systems/)

'Vanguard' sites (including new models of general practice)

As part of the NHS *Five Year Forward View* and NHS England's new care models programme, 50 'vanguard' sites are seeking to develop new ways of working, accelerate improvements in care and share lessons learned with other areas and with national policy makers.

According to NHS England there are five vanguard types:

- *Integrated primary and acute care systems* – *joining up GP, hospital, community and mental health services*
- *Multispecialty community providers* – *moving specialist care out of hospitals into the community*
- *Enhanced health in care homes* – *offering older people better, joined up health, care and rehabilitation services*
- *Urgent and emergency care* – *new approaches to improve the coordination of services and reduce pressure on A&E departments*
- *Acute care collaborations* – *linking local hospitals together to improve their clinical and financial viability, reducing variation in care and efficiency. (NHS England, Models of care, www. england.nhs.uk/new-care-models/about/)*

Summaries of each site and regular updates are available via the NHS England website.

In many areas of the country, new models of general practice are also developing – with local GP surgeries working together to cover much larger patient populations and to provide more comprehensive care, either through a 'super-partnership' (where practices merge into one entity) or a 'federation' (where practices retain their independence, but have a collaborative agreement with other practices).

Job satisfaction, stress and care as emotional labour

For many people working in health and social care, the contribution they make is one of the greatest privileges there is – on a good day, it's hard to imagine anything that matters more or that can be more rewarding. Equally, many roles are very pressured, involve significant human distress and the stakes are as high as they can be if something goes wrong – in many ways, it's also hard to imagine any jobs that could be harder. Anyone who wants to work in health and social care therefore needs to think about what motivates them, what they enjoy and what they're good at – as well as about ways of managing stress, remaining compassionate and staying healthy oneself.

In the NHS, an annual staff survey has been conducted since 2003 and is thought to be the largest workforce survey in the world (see **Facts and Figures 11** for a summary of the 2017 results). There is also a quarterly staff version of the **Friends and Family Test**, whereby staff are asked whether they would recommend their service to their own friends or families if they were unwell and needed support, or as a place to work. Between July and September 2017, some 137,225 people took part:

- 80% would recommend their organisation to a friend or family member, with 14% responding 'neither/don't know' and 6% not recommending.
- 63% would recommend their organisation as a place to work, with 19% not recommending and 18% responding 'neither/don't know'. (NHS England, Staff Friends and Family Test, Quarter 2 2017–18, www.england.nhs.uk/wp-content/uploads/2017/11/fft-staff-summary-q2-17-18.pdf)

While adult social care has data on staff turnover, vacancies and sickness rates, the social care system is essentially local and there is less systematic, national data available about staff morale. However, as outlined in Chapter Two, there are significant concerns about the stability and well-being of the social care workforce and significant criticism of government for the absence of an up-to-date adult social care workforce strategy (NAO, 2018).

Facts and Figures 11: NHS staff survey

According to NHS England:

The 2017 NHS Staff Survey is published today showing that staff feel under pressure but say they are being better supported by their NHS managers.

Overall staff engagement is scored 3.78 out of 5 in 2017, up from 3.68 out of 5 in 2012.

More than four out of five, 81%, are satisfied with the quality of care they give to patients and nine out of ten staff feel their organisation takes positive action on health and well-being.

Among the areas of concern highlighted by the research is that almost one in six members of staff, 15%, report that they have experienced physical violence from patients, relatives or members of the public.

The number satisfied with their pay fell to 31% down 6% on 2016.

Around a third of staff, 38%, said that they had experienced work related stress over the last 12 months, up 1.6% on the previous year but slightly down on five years ago.

Some 8% of staff say they have experienced discrimination from colleagues.

However, the number who said they were happy with the support they receive from their manager increased for the fifth year in a row to almost seven out of 10 (68%). Fewer staff also feel pressured by managers or colleagues to come to work when they are ill and fewer staff are working unpaid hours.

The survey was carried out in the run up to and during the NHS' pressurised winter between September and December 2017 across 309 NHS organisations garnering 485,000 staff responses, an increase of 64,000 and an increase of 21% in responses from BME [black and minority ethnic] staff. This takes in views from about a third of the NHS workforce and is the biggest response achieved in the survey's 15-year history.

Source: NHS England, www.england.nhs.uk/2018/03/nhs-england-publishes-latest-nhs-staff-survey-results

One of the key ways in which we could improve services and better support staff is to recognise the unique nature of care. As Sawbridge and Hewison (2011; see also Hewison and Sawbridge, 2016) have argued, care work is difficult, distressing and quite often fairly disgusting (involving bodily functions and fluids that we wouldn't often talk about in open, polite conversation). To deal with so much pain, distress and even death, workers need to feel really supported in what they do – otherwise it can be very difficult to keep going and to retain your humanity in the face of so much suffering (see **Voices of Experience 12**). In this sense, care is a form of **emotional labour** – we all have an 'emotional bank account' that gets depleted by the horrible things we see in health and social care, and we all have to find ways of topping up that bank account to stay in credit (healthy, well, happy, fulfilled). Too often, large health and social care organisations (and their leaders) find themselves having to focus on money, on performance data, on government 'must dos' and on regulatory interventions. These are all important, but they can also distract from the fundamental task of appointing people with the right skills and values to look after people in significant distress, and to support those staff to deliver high quality, dignified, person-centred care, day in and day out. All the available evidence suggests that it is very difficult to deliver good care if you don't feel supported yourself (see, for example, West et al, 2017), and yet staff support often feels like a low priority (or something to which we only really pay lip service). While NHS Boards or local authority committees might sometimes say that 'staff are our greatest resource', do we really follow this through when it comes to drawing up our priorities? It can be really instructive to watch a Board or Committee meeting (many are now open to the public, and some are live-streamed). How many times does the Board mention money and targets, compared to how many times it mentions staff well-being?

Looking at what happens when something goes really wrong in health and social care, Sawbridge and Hewison have tried to shift the emphasis away from finding an individual to blame. While individuals may have made mistakes (or sometimes even done something negligent or criminal in nature), we often find that the broader environment and culture has somehow lost sight of the care it is meant to be providing, and that staff have become ground down by what they have to see and do, without adequate support. They have therefore been running projects with a series of nurse leaders to look at different ways of supporting staff, and have even worked with the Samaritans (comparing how they support volunteers to do such distressing work with how the NHS supports (or often fails to support) its nurses and care workers). While the former Chair of the health and social care regulator in England was quoted as saying that "giving someone a smile costs nothing", Sawbridge and Hewison have argued this is true financially – but is not true emotionally (and is a fundamental misunderstanding of the nature of care). As they observe, you may be at the end of a 12-hour shift and be cleaning up an older person with dementia who has soiled themselves and become really distressed. You try to do this as compassionately as possible, but it's not very nice, you're exhausted and the situation reminds you of your own mother who died with dementia. You therefore take yourself off to clean up in the sluice room (often the only private space) and for a quiet cry – then you come back onto the ward to look after the person in the next bed along, as if they were the only person on the ward. Giving someone a smile costs nothing financially – but it costs an awful lot in other ways, and we neglect this at our peril.

Voices of Experience 12: Care as emotional labour

"I am in charge tonight with five nurses and 30 patients. Two of my nurses are floats who have never been on the floor; one will be an hour late, so I will have to cover her patients. Our medical-surgical patients have diagnoses (including) failure of the kidney, stroke, diabetes, cancer, sickle cell disease, hepatitis, AIDs, pneumonia and Alzheimer's disease.

The average age of our patients is 79. We have five fresh post-operative patients and one going to surgery in two hours. As I come out of report one of our stable patients who transferred from Coronary Care Unit yesterday, is having chest pain. There is a Dr on the phone waiting to give admission orders and the anaesthetist for our pre-operative patient wants the old chart, now. Down the hall an elderly confused patient has just crawled over the side rails and fallen. Two of our fresh post-op patients, are vomiting as a side effect of the anaesthesia, (and) their families are very tense and need reassuring. One of the patients I am covering for has just pulled out his IV; another wants something for pain; another needed the bed pan and I got there too late. The lab has called with a critical low haemoglobin level on the patient who pulled out his IV; he'll be getting a few units of blood as soon as possible.

This condensed version represents the first two hours of my working day ... it is no fabrication." (Benner and Wrubel, 1989, p 365)

"Staff don't need more blame and condemnation; they need active, sustained supervision and support. In the high-volume, high-pressure, complex environment of modern health care it is very difficult to remain sensitive and caring towards every single patient all of the time. We ask ourselves how it is possible that anyone, let alone a nurse, could ignore a dying man's request for water? What we should also ask is whether it is humanly possible for anyone to look after very sick, very frail, possibly incontinent,

possibly confused patients without excellent induction, training, supervision and support." (Cornwell, 2011)

Source: Sawbridge and Hewison's (2011) policy paper on emotional labour.

The two quotes are over 20 years apart, suggesting that we have known about these issues for some time.

Skills and training

Another way of responding to all the challenges and changes summarised in this book is to have high quality training and support, and then to keep updating one's skills and knowledge over time. Without this, there is a danger that we qualify with a particular set of skills and in a particular context, but that our ability to provide good care is diminished by acquiring bad habits in practice and/or by failing to keep pace with changing technology, new evidence and ideas, developments in other sectors and a rapidly changing policy context. Keeping up-to-date can also be crucial for people in senior leadership roles (and when researching and teaching within universities), as it's easy to think that we understand the realities of frontline services, only to discover that the world has moved on since we trained or last looked. With this in mind, both health and social care have a strong commitment to ongoing training and development (albeit it can sometimes be difficult to release staff when services are under pressure, or if training budgets are cut). Indeed, this can be a significant attraction to staff, with a series of different opportunities for people at different stages of their careers. This might include:

- Apprenticeships and training on-the-job;
- Professional training courses needed to become a doctor, nurse, social worker, OT, physio or other health and social professional;
- Training provided by employers, including mandatory training (around topics such as manual handling, information governance, child protection or infection control);

- National frameworks and resources provided by sector skills councils (see **Key Sources 13** for an adult social care example);
- Specialist postgraduate qualifications;
- Leadership development opportunities (at all levels of seniority) (see, for example, **Voices of Experience 8** in Chapter Five).

Key Sources 13: Learning and development in adult social care

Everyone working in adult social care should be able to take part in learning and development so they can carry out their role effectively. This will help to develop the right skills and knowledge so you can provide high quality care and support.

In this section of the website you'll find information and resources to help with the 'Care Certificate', the minimum standards that should be covered as part of induction.

To ensure you have a capable, confident and skilled workforce you should continue to develop staff beyond induction.

Find out about the flexible qualifications and apprenticeships available to meet the different needs of your workforce.

We can help fund related training and adult social care qualifications. Our funding pages provide information on what's available.

If you need support finding and choosing the right learning we have a practical guide to help. You should also take a look at our 'learning provider directory' that details all the providers who are part of our 'Endorsement Framework' and have been given our mark of quality.

Our leadership development programmes are perfect for people in top roles in social care who want to improve their skills and meet other people working in similar roles.

If you work with newly qualified social workers we have tools to help you implement the 'Assessed and Supported Year in Employment (ASYE)' [12 month programme to support and assess newly qualified social workers] in adults and child and family services. We also have resources to help with the continuing professional development of social workers.

Take a look at our 'core skills guide' to help develop the English, number, digital and employability skills of your staff. These skills will underpin all learning and development activity.

Our guide to On-going learning and development in adult social care can help you to create and keep a knowledgeable, skilled and up-to-date workforce.

Source: Learning and Development, Skills for Care, www.skillsforcare. org.uk/Learning-development/Learning-and-development.aspx

The future workforce and seven day services

As suggested at various stages throughout this book, the health and social care workforce is under significant pressure – and different governments over time have found it hard to plan ahead to meet future workforce needs and to prevent potentially significant gaps and staff shortages. This is partly because our political system operates on a relatively short-term basis (with elections every five years), while the time taken to train and develop a new and then a senior clinician is much longer. For example, it takes around 10 years to train as a GP and 14 years to train as a surgeon, so any government that identified a potential shortage of these workers today would be unable to resolve the problem by training more people for a significant period of time.

Faced with these realities, there have been a number of debates over time about how best to ensure an appropriate workforce, including:

- *Recruiting qualified and experienced workers from abroad* (where their training and qualifications are consistent with UK standards): while this can provide new staff relatively quickly, this deprives the person's country of origin of skilled workers, and new staff working in the UK may need significant support to acclimatise (for example, if they are relocating from a different country, leaving family behind and/or improving their language skills). Some workers who come to the UK also report experiencing racism, whether from patients, colleagues or outside work.
- *Exploring scope for new roles* that blur the boundaries of traditional professions, or that enable current staff to take on new skills: examples of this may include roles such as physician associates, nurses taking a greater role in prescribing medication or consultant paramedics. While this can be really positive, it can also raise questions about how best to train and support people and create tensions with existing roles.

At the time of writing, a significant unknown is the impact of Brexit and an apparent hardening of public and political attitudes to immigration (see **Facts and Figures 12**). While the long-term implications of this are unknown, UK health and social care have always relied on migration, with both sectors benefitting tremendously from the skills and experience of international staff choosing to come and work in the UK. Although these issues have acquired recent prominence, this has always been the case – dating back at least as far as the 1950s, when there were recruitment campaigns to persuade Caribbean nurses to come to the UK to practise. According to a summary by the King's Fund (McKenna, 2017), nearly 62,000 (5.6%) of the English NHS's workforce and an estimated 95,000 (around 7%) of England's adult social care workforce are people who have come to work in the UK from other EU countries:

Recent estimates suggest that both the health and social care sectors will face a considerable shortfall in staff in future if EU migration is limited after Brexit. Modelling from Department of Health published in the HSJ [*Health Service Journal*] projects (under a worst case scenario) a shortage in the UK of between 26,000 to 42,000 nurses (full-time equivalents) by 2025/26 ... Projections from the Nuffield Trust suggest a shortfall in England of as many as 70,000 social care workers (headcount) by the same date.

Moreover, there are a large number of older people (some becoming frailer over time) who currently live in Brittany and parts of Spain, and there remain significant uncertainties about their future status and about what might happen if those people were not able to access care in their current place of residence or if a significant number of these people chose to come back to the UK at the same time. This is also creating anxiety and uncertainty for the individuals concerned. As but one example, the University of Birmingham has worked with the British Consulate in Malaga to set up a new website (www.supportinspain.info) that provides a directory of support services and a list of helpful topics (how to access health and social care, becoming resident in Spain, benefits and financial advice) for older UK nationals with care needs living in Spain.

Facts and Figures 12: Brexit and the international make-up of health and social care staff

In terms of social care, the charity Independent Age, estimates that:

- *Around 1 in 20 (6%) of England's growing social care workforce are EEA migrants, equating to around 84,000 people. Further, more than 90% of those EEA migrants (78,000) do not have British citizenship – meaning they could be at risk of changes to their immigration status following Brexit.*
- *In a zero net migration scenario, the social care workforce gap could reach just above 1.1 million workers by 2037. This means that there would be 13.5 older people for every care worker – compared to a ratio of seven for every care worker today. This is a workforce gap which, by 2037, is around 70,000 workers larger than our worst predictions in our analysis pre-EU referendum.*
- *In a (more likely) low-migration scenario, where the sector remains as attractive as it is today, but the government delivers on its commitment to reduce levels of net migration, there will be a social care workforce gap of more than 750,000 people by 2037.*
- *Even in a scenario where there are high levels of migration and the care sector becomes more attractive, the social care gap will be as big as 350,000 people by 2037. The implications of a social care workforce gap of between 350,000 and 1.1 million workers for older and disabled people are clear – far fewer will be able to access the care they need to live meaningful, independent lives. (www. independentage.org/policy-and-research/research-reports/ brexit-and-future-of-migrants-social-care-workforce)*

In the NHS, the House of Commons Library has highlighted the international nature of the NHS workforce:

Around 139,000 out of 1.2 million NHS staff report a non-British nationality (12.5% of all staff for whom a nationality is known, or one in every eight). Between them, these staff hold 200 different non-British nationalities. Around 62,000 are nationals of other EU countries – 5.6% of NHS staff in England. Around 47,000 staff are Asian nationals. (https://researchbriefings.parliament.uk/ResearchBriefing/Summary/CBP-7783)

Of every 1,000 NHS staff in England, 875 are British, 56 are from other EU countries, 42 are Asian, 19 are African and 8 are from somewhere else.

Most common nationalities of NHS staff

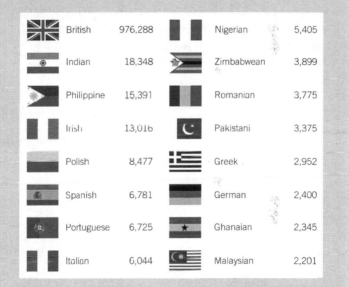

British	976,288		Nigerian	5,405
Indian	18,348		Zimbabwean	3,899
Philippine	15,391		Romanian	3,775
Irish	13,016		Pakistani	3,375
Polish	8,477		Greek	2,952
Spanish	6,781		German	2,400
Portuguese	6,725		Ghanaian	2,345
Italian	6,044		Malaysian	2,201

Source: https://researchbriefings.parliament.uk/ResearchBriefing/Summary/CBP-7783

A final delivery challenge concerns ongoing debates about the types of care we should be providing at different times of the day and on different days of the week (often described as a debate around 'seven day services'). This became very controversial in 2015–16, as the Conservatives committed to make England 'the first country in the world to provide a truly seven day service' (Conservative Party, 2015, p 38). Later on, there were attempts to remodel medical contracts to make late evenings and Saturdays a part of the normal working week, culminating in strike action by junior doctors. Particularly controversial were claims that hospitals were less safe at weekends with fewer senior staff leading to harm to patients. In contrast, opponents of these proposed changes argued that the issue at stake was about pay (normal hours v extra payments for anti-social hours) and not about quality. Subsequent research has also suggested that the picture is much more complex, and that governments should be wary of drawing a causal relationship between staffing and the so-called 'weekend effect' (for example, it may be that people admitted at the weekend are sicker than during the week, so that mortality might be expected to be higher). Others have pointed out that NHS staff typically work many more hours than those for which they are paid (known as 'donated labour') and that contractual reform can often have unintended consequences – for example, if a new contract was imposed and people genuinely worked to the contract, then we may have even more shortages. Certainly there are key issues here – about which services we always need available 24/7 and in which locations; how we best balance the needs of patients and of staff; what kinds of social care support we need outside traditional office hours; and what kinds of diagnostic services we want, both now and in the future. However, at a time when funding is tight and when there are serious workforce shortages, this doesn't feel like the right debate to be having – and certainly not in such a controversial and polarised way. As Julian Bion, a leading researcher in this area, has argued:

> I'm convinced seven-day services cannot be achieved within current funding. There are huge gaps [in medical staffing rotas in hospitals already]. I think we're 20 years away from actually being

able to achieve a seven-day service given the current challenges, but I would love to be wrong. (quoted in Campbell, 2016)

Further resources

The King's Fund (2011) *Commission on Leadership and Management in the NHS* is available to download free of charge, challenging media stereotypes of the NHS as 'over-managed'.

Resources to support **new models of care** are provided by NHS England (www.england.nhs.uk/new-care-models/).

Information on the **NHS staff survey** and the **Staff Friends and Family Test** is available via www.nhsstaffsurveys.com/Page/1056/Home/NHS-Staff-Survey-2018/ and www.england.nhs.uk/fft/staff-fft/data/. The NAO (2018) has published a critical review of approaches to understanding and supporting the **adult social care workforce**.

Hewison and Sawbridge's work on **care as emotional labour** forms the basis of an edited book (2016) on *Compassion in Nursing*. An overview of these ideas is available as a TEDx talk on *Why Good People Might Deliver Bad Care* (www.youtube.com/watch?v=VC4FajTFpRU) and via a free online policy paper, *Time to Care?* (Sawbridge and Hewison, 2011).

Resources around **skills and training** are available via bodies such as:

- Health Education England (www.healthcareers.nhs.uk)
- Skills for Care (www.skillsforcare.org.uk)
- Skills for Health (www.skillsforhealth.org.uk)

Briefings on the implications of **Brexit** are provided by:

- Independent Age (www.independentage.org/policy-and-research/research-reports/brexit-and-future-of-migrants-social-care-workforce)
- The House of Commons Library (https://researchbriefings.parliament.uk/ResearchBriefing/Summary/CBP-7783)

- The King's Fund (www.kingsfund.org.uk/publications/articles/
  brexit-implications-health-social-care)
- The Nuffield Trust (www.nuffieldtrust.org.uk/research/
  brexit-relationship-eu-shape-nhs)

Debates around **seven day services** and/or resources for
implementing this policy aspiration are available via:

- NHS Improvement (https://improvement.nhs.uk/resources/
  seven-day-services)
- NHS England (www.england.nhs.uk/seven-day-hospital-services/)
- The British Medical Association (www.bma.org.uk/collective-
  voice/policy-and-research/nhs-structure-and-delivery/
  seven-day-services/show-us-your-plan)
- Academic studies such as the HiSLAC (High-intensity Specialist
  Led Acute Care) project (www.hislac.org)

Short summary and key messages

This book has sought to provide a short guide to health and social care for people interested in learning about and/or working in the NHS or adult social services (or who are interested as voters, taxpayers and citizens).

Among a number of topics, some of the key themes throughout the book include:

- The fundamental importance of health and social care – personally, politically and economically;
- The significance of history and of society, with current services shaped by a series of compromises over time and by the broader social, economic and cultural climate;
- Different ways of funding services and the impact this has on the way care is delivered;
- Different ways of organising services – and the tensions which reforms and reorganisations over time have sought to reconcile;
- The need to work across boundaries to meet needs in a more joined-up, coordinated way;
- The need to understand individuals, their families and communities in order to be able to provide good care;
- The key roles played by health and social care professionals, and the tremendous power and responsibility that comes with being a professional;
- The complexities and realities of delivering care – and the need for excellent staff support in order to enable frontline workers to deliver good care to others;
- The incredible pressures faced by both health and social care as they celebrate their 70th anniversaries.

However, while they are a time for reflection and for taking stock, anniversaries are mainly a time for celebration. To illustrate the importance of the issues at stake, this book ends with a series of stories shared by different individuals reflecting on what health and social care have meant to them and their families:

1. In 2008, Aneira Thomas, the first person to be born after the creation of the NHS (and named after Aneurin Bevan) was interviewed for the BBC to mark the 60th anniversary of the NHS.
2. In 2015, a celebration of 20 years of the Disability Discrimination Act published the memories and contributions of leading disability rights campaigners such as John Evans (who moved out of residential care in Hampshire in the 1980s and became an internationally recognised campaigner for disability rights and a pioneer of direct payments) and Baroness Jane Campbell (a member of the former Disability Rights Commission and independent Peer).
3. In 2014, the writer and political commentator, Harry Smith, addressed the Labour Party conference, remembering what life before the welfare state was like.

Voices of Experience 13: The first NHS baby

When Aneira Thomas's mother went into labour, the nurses pleaded with her to wait until the clock struck midnight. Both mother and child obliged – and a minute past the hour, on 5 July 1948, the first NHS baby was born at Amman Valley Hospital, Carmarthenshire. Naming the newborn was straightforward, the inspiration was the founding father of the NHS, Aneurin Bevan.

Sixty-years later, Mrs Thomas has kicked off celebrations to mark the foundation of Britain's health service. Visiting the modern maternity unit at Singleton Hospital in Swansea, she proudly handed out "Born in Wales" bibs to new mothers. "As a child I never understood what the significance of it was," admitted Mrs

Thomas ... "I just kept saying I was the first national health baby and didn't understand what it meant." For her mother Edna, who spent 18 hours in labour before giving birth, it meant no longer having to shell out the one shilling and sixpence in midwifery fees. For Edna's husband Willie, that would have made a serious dent in the £2 a week wages he earned as a miner down the Great Mountain pit in Tumble ...

Mrs Thomas forged a life-long link with the health service becoming a mental health nurse, along with her three sisters, and her daughter is now an ambulance technician. Her own life has been saved on two occasions when she had to be revived after suffering severe allergic reactions.

"The last one was near fatal," she said.

Sixty-years on, Mrs Thomas remains fiercely proud of the NHS, even as she admitted herself that there was always room for improvement. "There are lots of issues that should be addressed," she stated ... "But on the whole I think we are very, very, fortunate." (BBC, 2008)

Voices of Experience 14: Independent living

For me, Independent Living was the real liberation of disabled people from institutions and settings that were restricting inclusion into society.

Two key principles of independence were control and choice. We believed that rehabilitation, medical and social care experts shouldn't be making fundamental decisions about the lives of disabled people.

The motto 'nothing about us without us' summed up the movement well. I started one of the first independent living schemes in the country. A group of us were living at Le Court Residential Cheshire Home in Hampshire and wanted to leave the institution.

Making choices

Along with seven other people I began to assert control over the decisions affecting my life and making choices. The law at the time was a problem. A local authority directly paid the residential home of the individual, not the individual themselves. We developed a solution which involved the indirect payment to the individual.

Our thinking was this: why should the local authority go on paying the residential home? Instead they should transfer the money into an individual's bank account so we could control our own budget and pay our own personal assistants.

We negotiated a financial agreement with the residential home which led to us moving out of the institution and living independently in the community. This marked the beginning of the Independent Living Movement in the UK.

This loophole worked in some areas, but other disabled people wanting Independent Living did not live in residential care. As some local authorities would not accept that transferring money to the individual was legal, they wouldn't take the risk.

Changing the law

In order to change the law to make Independent Living schemes available to all, we set up an Independent Living Committee inside the British Council of Organisations of Disabled People (BCODP), the umbrella organisation of groups run by, not just for, disabled people. Our goal was to ensure direct payments would be made to everybody wanting them.

At the same time, we set up the first Centres of Independent Living to share our experiences and build our campaigning. We set up the Hampshire Centre for Independent Living in 1984, which was the first of its kind in the UK along with Derbyshire

Centre for Integrated Living and later the Greenwich Centre for Independent Living.

John Evans OBE, SCOPE campaign for independent living, 4 Nov 2015 (https://blog.scope.org.uk/2015/11/04/fighting-for-independent-living-dda20/)

All throughout my segregated school days, where I was taught nothing apart from how to cook cheese on toast, make pottery vases and learn about dinosaurs, my life was in black and white. At 16 I could just about read and write and add up. I was acutely aware of the difference between me and my sister, who went to an ordinary school and got to do all the things that I wanted to do.

It was only when I went away to university that life began to turn into colour. I began to feel liberated because I started to learn. I learnt academically and I learnt socially.

It was hard because barriers to my participation were everywhere but at least I was present. I joined various uni-societies, as much as I physically could, and became an active member of the 'Feminism Soc'.

I was a women's rights activist long before a disability one. My Master's degree dissertation focused on the suffragette Sylvia Pankhurst who organised working women's suffrage campaigns.

If I could go back in time, she's the woman I would want to be. I wanted a moment of liberation exactly like Sylvia Pankhurst had achieved. I wanted to be part of bringing about a legal watershed moment, just like she did. Little did I know then that this time would come.

Changing society

An early lesson for me was that nothing would change without a mass movement to infiltrate every part of society and demand change. We came up with a saying in the disability movement – "nothing about us without us". This means having a mandate to change society, so it would comply with the Social Model of Disability.

To do that, we needed to involve all disabled people in our movement, not just people in wheelchairs who dominated at the beginning. That was quite a challenge because we had to deal with our own prejudices about other impairments.

I've always been struck by how collective the disability movement was and how mutually supportive we were when organising our campaigns. I think we did more than most civil rights groups to ensure that all of our activities were as accessible as they could be so everyone could join in.

Getting arrested

I wasn't afraid to test the law. I would be found in the middle of the street with my disabled brothers and sisters. People who used electric wheelchairs were very useful because the one thing about an electric chair is that you cannot lift one without putting out your back!

In the early days of the civil rights campaign, it was impossible to get arrested, try as we might. The police didn't know whether to pat us on the head, give us a pound, or arrest us. They were so confused. They couldn't get disabled people into their meat wagons, if they managed to get us to a police station, there were no accessible toilets or cells.

I remember police officers taking wheelchair users they had arrested across the road to an accessible toilet in a hotel and end up buying them a coffee, and then letting them go.

Liberation

All in all, my childhood of segregation, initiation into the Disability Movement and then the campaign for the DDA, was pretty much what made me the person I am today. I honestly wouldn't have had it any other way.

The law itself and the campaign were just small parts of what came out of taking part in our liberation struggle. The experience enabled me to understand who I really was and what I wanted. One of those things was politics, which eventually led me to enter Parliament as a Crossbencher in the House of Lords. And the rest, as they say, is history.

Baroness Jane Campbell, SCOPE blog, 5 November 2015 (https://blog.scope.org.uk/tag/dda20/?_ga=2.259618126.579992550.1539962871-1488848480.1539962871)

Voices of Experience 15: Life before the welfare state

Writer Harry Smith stole the show in Labour's debate on health and social care, reducing some delegates to tears as he recounted life before the NHS.

Ahead of a speech by shadow health secretary Andy Burnham, Mr Smith said his childhood was a "barbarous time".

"Rampant poverty and no healthcare were the norm of the Britain of my youth."

In a speech greeted with a standing ovation and widely praised on Twitter, he warned that the UK must "be vigilant" about the NHS.

"I came into this world in the rough and ready year of 1923," Mr Smith said. "I'm from Barnsley, and I can tell you that my

childhood, like so many others from that era, was not like an episode from Downton Abbey."

"Instead, it was a barbarous time, it was a bleak time, and it was an uncivilised time, because public health care didn't exist."

Hospitals, doctors and medicine were for "the privileged few, because they were run by profit", he said.

"My memories stretch back almost a hundred years, and if I close my eyes, I can smell the poverty that oozes from the dusty tenement streets of my boyhood," he added.

Mr Smith recalled the "anguished cries" of a woman dying from cancer who could not afford morphine, and how his eldest sister had wasted and died from tuberculosis at the age of ten, and was "dumped nameless into a pauper's pit".

His generation was "galvanised" after the Second World War to become "the tide that raised all boats", and his experiences led him to vote Labour and for the creation of the NHS in 1945.

"My heart is also with the people of the present, who because of welfare cuts and austerity measures are struggling once more to make ends meet, and whose futures I fear for," he added.

"Today, we must be vigilant, we must be vocal, we must demand that the NHS must always remain an institution for the people and by the people."

"We must never ever let the NHS free from our grasp, because if we do, your future will be my past."

BBC, 24 September 2014 (www.bbc.co.uk/news/uk-politics-29345395)

Running throughout these three examples are some key messages that no one associated with or interested in health and social care should forget:

- Life is inherently unpredictable, and any one of us could need services at any moment.
- Good quality health and social care transforms lives.
- While there are lots of challenges and things could always be better, we are incredibly lucky and have much to be thankful for.
- Whatever our current service and financial pressures, we do an amazing amount of good – and it's hard to imagine a greater privilege than to be part of something so special.
- These issues matter – and we all have a responsibility (as students, as workers, as researchers, as voters and taxpayers, as citizens) to find out more about and support our services if we want to keep them and improve them for the future.

References

Adams, R. (2010) *The Short Guide to Social Work*, Bristol: Policy Press.

Alakeson, V. (2014) *Delivering Personal Health Budgets: A guide to policy and practice*, Bristol: Policy Press.

Alcock, P., Haux, T., May, M. and Wright, S. (2016) *The Student's Guide to Social Policy* (5th ed.), Oxford: Wiley Blackwell.

Allen, K. and Glasby, J. (2010) *'The Billion Dollar Question': Embedding prevention in older people's services – 10 high impact changes*, Birmingham: Health Services Management Centre (Policy Paper 8).

Allen, K., Miller, R. and Glasby, J. (2013) *Prevention Services, Social Care and Older People: Much discussed but little researched?* London: School for Social Care Research (research findings summary).

Arnstein, S.R. (1969) A ladder of citizen participation, *Journal of the American Planning Association*, 35(4), 216–224.

Association of Directors of Adult Social Services (ADASS), ADASS Cymru, ADASS – Northern Ireland and Association of Directors of Social Work (ADSW) (2014) *Four Nations United: Critical learning from four different systems for the successful integration of social care and health services*, London: ADASS and ADSW.

Baggott, R. (2011) *Public Health Policy and Politics* (2nd ed.), Basingstoke: Palgrave Macmillan.

Baggott, R. (2013) *Partnerships for Public Health and Well-being*, Basingstoke: Palgrave Macmillan.

Barker, K. (2014) *A New Settlement for Health and Social Care*, London: King's Fund.

BBC News (2008) The birth of a baby and the NHS, 27 June, http://news.bbc.co.uk/1/hi/wales/7478283.stm

BBC (2014) Harry Smith, 91, brings tears to Labour delegates' eyes, 24 September, www.bbc.co.uk/news/uk-politics-29345395

Beauchamp, T.L. and Childress, J.E. (2012) *Principles of Biomedical Ethics* (7th ed.), Oxford: Oxford University Press (first edition published in 1979).

Benner, P. and Wrubel, J. (1989) *The Primacy of Caring: Stress and coping in health and illness*, Menlo Park, CA: Addison-Wesley.

Bevan, A. (1946) Speech on the Second Reading of the National Health Service Bill, *House of Commons Debates*, 30 April, vol 422, cc43–142, http://hansard.millbanksystems.com/commons/1946/apr/30/national-health-service-bill

Bevan, A. (1952) *In Place of Fear*, London: Heinemann.

Bevan, G., Karanikolos, M., Exley, J., Nolte, E., Connolly, S. and Mays, N. (2014) *The Four Health Systems of the United Kingdom: How do they compare?* London: Health Foundation/Nuffield Trust.

Bochel, H. and Powell, M. (eds) (2016) *The Coalition Government and Social Policy*, Bristol: Policy Press.

British Association of Social Workers (2014) *The Code of Ethics for Social Work: Statement of principles*, Birmingham: BASW.

Campbell, D. (2016) Seven-day NHS unachievable for 20 years, expert claims, *Guardian*, 18 July, www.theguardian.com/society/2016/jul/18/seven-day-nhs-unachievable-for-20-years-expert-claims

Care Quality Commission (2017) *The State of Health Care and Adult Social Care in England 2016/17*, London: CQC.

Carpenter, J. (1995) Doctors and nurses: stereotypes and stereotype change in interprofessional education, *Journal of Interprofessional Care*, 9(2), 151–161.

Carpenter, J. and Dickinson, H. (2016) *Interprofessional Education and Training* (2nd ed.), Bristol: Policy Press.

Chanan, G. and Fisher, B. (2018) *Commissioning Community Development for Health: A concise handbook*, London: Coalition for Collaborative Care, www.healthempowerment.co.uk/wp-content/uploads/2018/01/COMMISSIONING-CD-FOR-HEALTH-C4CC-2018-1.pdf

Colombo, F., LLena-Nozel, A., Mercier, J. and Tjadens, F. (2011) *Help Wanted?: Providing and paying for long-term care*, Paris, OECD Publishing, http://dx.doi.org/10.1787/9789264097759-en

Conradie, L. and Golding, T. (2013) *The Short Guide to Working with Children and Young People*, Bristol: Policy Press.

Conservative Party (2015) *The Conservative Party Manifesto 2015*, www.conservatives.com/manifesto2015

Cornwell, J. (2011) *Care and Compassion in the NHS*, London: King's Fund, www.kingsfund.org.uk/blog/2011/02/care-and-compassion-nhs-patient-experience

Crisp, N. (2011) *24 Hours to Save the NHS*, Oxford: Oxford University Press.

de Medeiros, K. (2016) *The Short Guide to Aging and Gerontology*, Bristol: Policy Press.

Department of Health (1998) *Partnership in Action: New opportunities for joint working between health and social services – a discussion document*, London: DH.

Dickinson, H. and Glasby, J. (2006) *Free Personal Care in Scotland*, London: King's Fund.

Dickinson, H., Glasby, J., Forder, J. and Beesley, L. (2007) Free personal care in Scotland: a narrative review, *British Journal of Social Work*, 37(1), 459–474.

Dilnot, A. (2011) *Fairer Care Funding*, London: Commission on Funding of Care and Support.

Edwards, N. (2010) *The Triumph of Hope over Experience: Lessons from the history of reorganisation*, London: NHS Confederation.

Esping-Andersen, G. (1990) *The Three Worlds of Welfare Capitalism*, Cambridge: Polity Press.

Exworthy, M., Mannion, R. and Powell, M. (eds) (2016) *Dismantling the NHS? Evaluating the impact of health reforms*, Bristol: Policy Press.

Foster, L., Brunton, A., Deeming, C. and Haux, T. (eds) (2015) *In Defence of Welfare 2*, Bristol: Policy Press/Social Policy Association.

General Medical Council (2014) *Good Medical Practice*, London: GMC.

Glasby, J. (ed) (2012) *Commissioning for Health and Well-being*, Bristol: Policy Press.

Glasby, J. (2016) *Understanding Health and Social Care* (3rd ed.), Bristol: Policy Press.

Glasby, J. and Dickinson, H. (2014) *Partnership Working in Health and Social Care* (2nd ed.), Bristol: Policy Press.

Glasby, J. and Littlechild, R. (2016) *Direct Payments and Personal Budgets: Putting personalisation into practice* (3rd ed.), Bristol: Policy Press.

Glasby, J. and Tew, J. (2015) *Mental Health Policy and Practice* (3rd ed.), Basingstoke, Palgrave Macmillan.

Glasby, J., Peck, E., Ham, C. and Dickinson, H. (2007) *'Things Can Only Get Better?'– The argument for NHS independence*, Birmingham: Health Services Management Centre.

Glasby, J., Miller, R. and Lynch, J. (2013) *'Turning the Welfare State Upside Down?': Developing a new adult social care offer*, Birmingham: Health Services Management Centre (policy paper 15), www.birmingham.ac.uk/Documents/college-social-sciences/social-policy/HSMC/publications/PolicyPapers/policy-paper-fifteen.pdf

Greener, I. (2008) *Healthcare in the UK*, Bristol: Policy Press.

Greener, I. (2018) No 18: History shows that more funding, not reorganisations, make the NHS better for us all, Social Policy Association 50th Anniversary Blog Series, www.social-policy.org.uk/50-for-50/funding-not-reorgnisations/

Ham, C. (2009) *Health Policy in Britain* (6th ed.), Basingstoke, Palgrave Macmillan.

Ham, C., Heenan, D., Longley, M. and Steel, D.R. (2013) *Integrated Care in Northern Ireland, Scotland and Wales: Lessons for England*, London: King's Fund.

Heenan, D. and Birrell, D. (2018) *The Integration of Health and Social Care in the UK*, Basingstoke: Palgrave Macmillan.

Hewison, A. and Sawbridge, Y. (eds) (2016) *Compassion in Nursing: Theory, evidence and practice*, Basingstoke: Palgrave Macmillan.

Hudson, B. (2016) The unsuccessful privatisation of social care: why it matters and how to curb it, LSE British Policy and Politics blog, 4 April, http://blogs.lse.ac.uk/politicsandpolicy/why-social-care-privatisation-is-unsuccessful/

Hudson, B. and Hardy, B. (2002) What is a 'successful' partnership and how can it be measured?, in C. Glendinning, M. Powell and K. Rummery (eds) *Partnerships, New Labour and the Governance of Welfare*, Bristol: Policy Press.

Hudson, J., Kühner, S. and Lowe, S. (2015) *The Short Guide to Social Policy* (2nd ed.), Bristol: Policy Press.

Hunter, D. (2016) *The Health Debate* (2nd ed.), Bristol: Policy Press.

Hunter, D. and Perkins, N. (2014) *Partnership Working in Public Health*, Bristol: Policy Press.

Hunter, D., Marks, L. and Smith, K. (2010) *The Public Health System in England*, Bristol: Policy Press.

Jack, S. (2017) The crisis: 10 years in three charts, BBC News, 9 August, www.bbc.co.uk/news/business-40869369

Jelphs, K., Dickinson, H. and Miller, R. (2016) *Working in Teams* (2nd ed.), Bristol: Policy Press.

Jones, L. (1994) *The Social Context of Health and Health Work*, Basingstoke: Palgrave.

Khurana, R., Nohria, N. and Penrice, D. (2005) Is business management a profession?, Harvard Business School, 21 February, https://hbswk.hbs.edu/item/is-business-management-a-profession

King's Fund (2011) *The Future of Leadership and Management in the NHS: No more heroes*, London: King's Fund.

King's Fund (2017) How the NHS is funded, 16 May, www.kingsfund.org.uk/projects/nhs-in-a-nutshell/how-nhs-funded

Klein, R. (2013) *The New Politics of the NHS* (7th ed.), London: Radcliffe Publishing.

Le Grand, J. (2003) *Motivation, Agency and Public Policy: Of knights and knaves, pawns and queens*, Oxford: Oxford University Press.

Le Grand, J. (2007) *The Other Invisible Hand: Delivering public services through choice and competition*, Princeton, NJ: Princeton University Press.

Le Grand, J. and Bartlett, W. (eds) (1993) *Quasi-markets and Social Policy*, Basingstoke: Macmillan.

Leutz, W. (1999) Five laws for integrating medical and social services: lessons from the United States and the United Kingdom, *The Milbank Quarterly*, 77(1), 77–110.

Marmot Review (2010) *Fair Society, Healthy Lives*, London: Marmot Review.

McKenna, H. (2017) Brexit: the implications for health and social care, London: King's Fund, 13 December, www.kingsfund.org.uk/publications/articles/brexit-implications-health-social-care

Means, R., Richards, S. and Smith, R. (2008) *Community Care: Policy and practice* (4th ed.), Basingstoke: Palgrave.

National Audit Office (NAO) (2014) *Adult Social Care in England: Overview*, London: NAO.

National Audit Office (NAO) (2018) *The Adult Social Care Workforce in England*, London: NAO.

Naylor, C. (2017) Is there 'parity of esteem' between mental and physical health? Big election questions, London, King's Fund, 19 May, www.kingsfund.org.uk/publications/articles/big-election-questions-parity-mental-physical-health

Needham, C. and Glasby, J. (eds) (2014) *Debates in Personalisation*, Bristol: Policy Press.

NHS (2015) *The NHS Constitution for England*, www.gov.uk/government/publications/the-nhs-constitution-for-england/the-nhs-constitution-for-england

NHS England (2014) *NHS Five Year Forward View*, Leeds: NHS England.

NHS England/Mental Health Taskforce (2016) *The Five Year Forward View for Mental Health*, Leeds: NHS England/Mental Health Taskforce.

NHS Support Federation (2017) *Time to End the Market Experiment in the NHS?* www.nhsforsale.info/contract-alert/contract-report-dec-2017.html

Nuffield Trust, Health Foundation and King's Fund (2017) *The Autumn Budget: Joint statement on health and social care*, London: Nuffield Trust/Health Foundation/King's Fund.

Nursing and Midwifery Council (2015) *Professional Standards of Practice and Behaviour for Nurses and Midwives*, London: NMC.

Nursing and Midwifery Council and General Medical Council (2012) *Joint Statement of Professional Values*, London: NMC/GMC.

Ouchi, W. and Johnson, A. (1978) Types of organisational control and their relationship to organisational well-being, *Administrative Science Quarterly*, 23, 292–317.

Payne, G. (ed) (2013) *Social divisions* (3rd ed.), Basingstoke: Palgrave Macmillan.

Peck, E. and Crawford, A. (2002) 'You say tomato': culture as a signifier of difference between health and social care, *Mental Health Review Journal*, 7(3), 23–26.

Peck, E. and Crawford, A. (2004) 'Culture' in partnerships – what do we mean by it and what can we do about it?, Leeds: Integrated Care Network.

Peckham, S., Exworthy, M., Powell, M. and Greener, I. (2005) *Decentralisation, Centralisation and Devolution in Publicly Funded Health Services: Decentralisation as an organisational model for health-care in England*, July, report for the National Co-ordinating Centre for NHS Service Delivery and Organisation.

Powell, M. (ed) (2007) *Understanding the Mixed Economy of Welfare*, Bristol: Policy Press.

Powell, M. (2015) Who killed the English National Health Service?, *International Journal of Health Policy and Management*, 24(5), 267–269.

Powell, M. (2018) Exploring 70 years of the British National Health Service through anniversary documents, *International Journal of Health Policy and Management*, doi 10.15171/ijhpm.2018.21.

Powell, M. and Miller, R. (2014) Framing privatisation in the English National Health Service, *Journal of Social Policy*, 43(3), 575–94.

Powell, M. and Miller, R. (2015) Seventy years of privatizing the British National Health Service?, *Social Policy and Administration*, 50(1), 99–118.

Robertson, R., Gregory, S. and Jabbal, J. (2014) *The Social Care and Health Systems of Nine Countries*, London: King's Fund.

Sawbridge, Y. (2016) Care closer to home – a fairytale?, Birmingham: Health Services Management Centre, www.birmingham.ac.uk/schools/social-policy/departments/health-services-management-centre/news/viewpoint/2016/10/care-closer-to-home-a-fairytale.aspx

Sawbridge, Y. and Hewison, A. (2011) *Time to Care? Responding to concerns about poor nursing care*, Birmingham: Health Services Management Centre.

SCIE (2017) *Asset-based Places: A model for development*, London: SCIE.

SCIE (2018) *Growing Innovative Models of Health, Care and Support for Adults*, London: SCIE.

Skills for Care (2017) *The State of the Adult Social Care Sector and Workforce in England, 2017*, Leeds: Skills for Care.

Sutherland, S. (1999) *With Respect to Old Age: Long term care – rights and responsibilities*, London: TSO.

Timmins, N. (2008) *Rejuvenate or Retire? Views on the NHS at 60*, London: Nuffield Trust.

Walshe, K. (2003) Foundation hospitals: a new direction for NHS reform?, *Journal of the Royal Society of Medicine*, 96, 106–110.

Wanless, D. (2006) *Securing Good Care for Older People: Taking a long-term view*, London: King's Fund.

Wenzel, L. (2018) *Approaches to Social Care Funding*, London: Health Foundation/King's Fund.

West, M. (2012) *Effective Teamwork: Practical lessons from organizational research* (3rd ed.), Oxford: Wiley Blackwell.

West, M., Eckert, R., Collins, B. and Chowla, R. (2017) *Caring to Change: How compassionate leadership can stimulate innovation in health care*, London: King's Fund.

WHO (2008) *Closing the Gap in a Generation: Health equity through action on the social determinants of health*, Geneva: WHO.

Index

Note: page numbers in *italic* type refer to further resources.